T0271875

Pass the MRCP (SCE) Neurology Revision Guide

This up-to-date revision guide for the MRCP SCE (Membership of the Royal College of Physicians—Specialty Certificate Examination) in neurology covers the core areas essential for exam success. The chapters are structured to align with the exam syllabus and help exam candidates learn and recall core concepts.

The chapter format and style provide a structured and focused approach to studying essential neurology topics, ensuring a comprehensive understanding of the subject matter. Carefully curated content encompasses all areas tested in the MRCP (SCE) Neurology examination. The use of bullet points, tables and colour illustrations aids in easy assimilation of information. The inclusion of neuroradiology and neuropathology, which account for a significant section of exam questions, is a particular strength of this text.

Whether you are a resident or trainee preparing for your first SCE examination or a seasoned neurologist seeking to enhance your knowledge and skills, this book will provide you with the necessary tools for success.

MasterPass Series

ENT OSCEs: A Guide to Your First ENT Job and Passing the MRCS (ENT) OSCE, 3E
Peter Kullar, Joseph Manjaly, Livy Kenyon

The Final FFICM Structured Oral Examination Study Guide
Eryl Davies

ENT Vivas: A Guide to Passing the Intercollegiate FRCS (ORL-HNS) Viva Examination
Adnan Darr, Karan Jolly, Jameel Muzaffar

Plastic Surgery Vivas for the FRCS (Plast): An Essential Guide
Monica Fawzy

Clinical Consultation Skills in Medicine: A Primer for MRCP PACES
Ernest Suresh

Neurosurgery: The Essential Guide to the Oral and Clinical Neurosurgical Exam, 2E
Vivian Elwell, Ramez Kirollos, Syed Al-Haddad, Peter Bodkin

Sport and Exercise Medicine: An Essential Guide
David Eastwood, Dane Vishnubala

Refraction and Retinoscopy: How to Pass the Refraction Certificate, 2E
Jonathan Park, Leo Feinberg, David Jones

Diagnostic EMQs: A Comprehensive Collection for Medical Examinations
Syed Hussain, Umber Rind, Jawed Noori, Yasmean Kalam, Haseeb Ata, Emanuel Papageorgiou

Postgraduate Ophthalmology Exam Success
Maneck Nicholson, Anjali Nicholson and Syed Faraaz Hussain

Cases in Haematology: For the MLA and PLAB
Aaron Niblock

Pass the MRCP (SCE) Neurology Revision Guide
Dhananjay Gupta

For more information about this series please visit: https://www.routledge.com/MasterPass/book-series/CRCMASPASS

Pass the MRCP (SCE) Neurology Revision Guide

Dhananjay Gupta

MBBS, MD (Medicine), DM (Neurology)
MRCP (SCE) Neurology
Fellowship in Stroke and Neuro-intervention

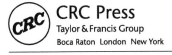

CRC Press
Taylor & Francis Group
Boca Raton London New York

CRC Press is an imprint of the
Taylor & Francis Group, an **informa** business

Cover image: Shutterstock ID 366499784

First edition published 2025
by CRC Press
6000 Broken Sound Parkway NW, Suite 300, Boca Raton, FL 33487–2742

and by CRC Press
4 Park Square, Milton Park, Abingdon, Oxon, OX14 4RN

CRC Press is an imprint of Taylor & Francis Group, LLC

© 2025 Dhananjay Gupta

Library of Congress Cataloging-in-Publication Data
Names: Gupta, Dhananjay (Neurologist), author.
Title: Pass the MRCP (SCE) neurology revision guide / Dhananjay Gupta. Other titles: Master pass.
Description: First edition. | Boca Raton, FL : CRC Press, 2024. | Series: Master pass | Includes bibliographical references and index.
Identifiers: LCCN 2024019526 (print) | LCCN 2024019527 (ebook) | ISBN 9781032433745 (hardback) | ISBN 9781032433738 (paperback) | ISBN 9781003367024 (ebook)
Subjects: MESH: Nervous System Diseases | Examination Questions
Classification: LCC RC343.5 (print) | LCC RC343.5 (ebook) | NLM WL 18.2 | DDC 616.80076—dc23/eng/20241015
LC record available at https://lccn.loc.gov/2024019526
LC ebook record available at https://lccn.loc.gov/2024019527

ISBN: 978-1-032-43374-5 (hbk)
ISBN: 978-1-032-43373-8 (pbk)
ISBN: 978-1-003-36702-4 (ebk)

DOI:10.1201/b23306

Typeset in Minion Pro
by Apex CoVantage, LLC

CONTENTS

PREFACE

The MRCP SCE (Specialty Certificate Examination) in Neurology is a pivotal milestone on the path to becoming a qualified consultant neurologist, showcasing the highest level of expertise in the field.

The first edition of this comprehensive revision book has been thoughtfully designed to assist physicians in their preparation for this demanding examination. It offers a structured and focused approach to studying essential neurology topics, ensuring a comprehensive understanding of the subject matter. The content within this book has been carefully curated to cover all the key areas tested in the MRCP SCE Neurology examination. The chapters are organized according to the syllabus of the examination and have been designed in the form of tables, figures and bullet points, which are easy to read and remember. Each chapter consists of concise yet comprehensive information, designed to help the reader master core concepts efficiently and effectively.

A standout feature of this book is the dedicated chapter on neuroradiology and neuropathology, which would account for 15–20% of the examination questions.

I hope that this MRCP SCE Neurology book proves to be an essential companion on your journey towards success in the examination. Whether you are a resident preparing for your first attempt or a seasoned neurologist seeking to enhance your knowledge and skills, I believe that this book will provide you with the necessary tools for success.

Best wishes for your MRCP SCE Neurology examination and for a rewarding career in neurology!

Dhananjay Gupta

AUTHOR

Dr. Dhananjay Gupta is a distinguished medical professional with a robust academic background and extensive clinical expertise in neurology. He completed his MBBS from the prestigious Vardhman Mahavir Medical College and Safdarjung Hospital, New Delhi, 2014. Subsequently, he pursued his MD (General Medicine) from PGI-MER and Dr. Ram Manohar Lohia Hospital, New Delhi. Further, he achieved his super-specialization in Neurology from MS Ramaiah Medical College, Bangalore, along with short-term training in neuropathology and neuroradiology from NIMHANS (National Institute of Mental Health and Neuro-Sciences), which is one of the best neuroscience research institutes in India.

Dr. Gupta's professional journey includes a clinical fellowship in stroke and neuro-interventional surgical procedures, enhancing his proficiency in managing complex neurological conditions. His commitment to advancing neurology is underscored by numerous publications in esteemed national and international journals, reflecting his scholarly contributions to the field. He has also presented papers and posters at various conferences earning accolades such as the Best Original Paper in Neurology and the Best Poster at the National Conference of Indian Academy of Neurology, held at Hyderabad in 2019.

Actively engaged in professional associations, Dr. Gupta is a member of both the Indian and the European Academy of Neurology. He plays an active role in activities of stroke and epilepsy associations around the country, contributing to research, education and advocacy in these critical areas of neurological practice. He is experienced in managing various neurological conditions like headache, neck pain, back pain and nerve and muscle diseases, and his areas of interest include neurological emergencies like stroke, epilepsy and autoimmune neurology.

Dr. Gupta's dedication to excellence in neurology, combined with his academic achievements and clinical acumen, makes him a valuable contributor to the medical community and a trusted resource for medical education and professional development in neurology.

CONTRIBUTORS

Haripriya Gupta, MBBS
Department of Neurology
Doaba Hospital and NeuroCare Centre
Jalandhar, India

Anuja Patel, BPT
Department of Neurology
Doaba Hospital and NeuroCare Centre
Jalandhar, India

CEREBROVASCULAR DISEASES

1. ATHEROSCLEROTIC CEREBROVASCULAR DISEASES: STROKE

Definition of Stroke (WHO, 1970): "Rapidly developing clinical signs of focal (or global) disturbance of cerebral function, lasting more than 24 hours or leading to death, with no apparent cause other than of vascular origin".

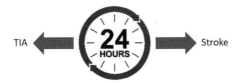

TIA ← **24 HOURS** → Stroke

Figure 1.1   Schematic representation of TIA and stroke.

We will highlight certain points or clues to look for in questions to identify a particular condition.

Table 1.1   Difference between Two Types of Watershed Infarctions

Cortical/External watershed zone stroke	Sub-cortical/Internal watershed stroke
More benign	More malignant/Poor prognosis
Pathogenesis: Hemodynamic factors are less common in pathogenesis of external watershed infarction More related to embolism from proximal source • Recent intra-plaque hemorrhage or plaque rupture in presence of ICA stenosis • Cortical watershed areas have less ability to "wash-out" emboli and less perfusion	Pathogenesis is more related to hemodynamic factors; in association with a proximal large artery stenosis
Imaging: Wedge-shaped or ovoid infarcts Infarcts are of variable sizes	Usually, 3 or more lesions adjacent to lateral ventricle Each 3 mm or more
Location depends on the variable distribution of ACA, MCA, PCA and the Lepto-meningeal collaterals	Located in a linear fashion parallel to the lateral ventricle in the corona radiata or centrum semi-ovale (rosary beads) Or cigar shaped
Extensive bilateral ACA/MCA: Man in barrel syndrome Proximal >> distal limb weakness	Brief hemodynamic compromise = Partial infarct Prolonged = Confluent infarct—step wise hemiplegia
Balint syndrome: Bilateral PCA/MCA watershed stroke Optic ataxia, oculomotor apraxia, dorsal simultangnosia	

DOI: 10.1201/b23306-1

	Disease	Clinical features	Neuroimaging
1.	**Watershed area stroke** hemodynamic factor related (see Table 1.1)	Risk factors of hypotension • Decrease in Blood Pressure • Post surgery patients • Acute Myocardial Infarction • Shock • Significant carotid stenosis Figure 1.2 MRI-DWI showing internal watershed infarcts.	These strokes are located in • **INTERNA**L watershed zone • B/W superficial and deep territories (perfusion) of MCA • Adjacent to lateral ventricle • Along the white matter • They spare the cortex • ROSARY BEADS sign
2.	**Locked-in syndrome**	A clinical presentation of: • Quadriplegia + aphasia + horizontal eye movements (EOM) palsy Only movements preserved are • Eye blinking • Vertical EOM because they are controlled by midbrain tectum Cause: Stroke: Infarct is located in Ventral pons (basis pontis) • Usually secondary to Basilar artery occlusion	 Figure 1.3 Axial MRI brain showing hyperintensities in ventral pons and right cerebellum. The patient presented in a locked-in state.
3.	Abulia	**Abulia** with or without confusion	Due to a Right caudate stroke
4.	Abulia	With right-side weakness	Due to a Left caudate + left putamen stroke

Table 1.2 Cause of Stroke in Autoimmune Diseases

In acute stage	In long term
More likely in young patients Exacerbation of disease (eg IBD) High inflammatory markers (ESR, CRP) Related to coagulopathy Hyper-coagulable state	High CRP Pro-inflammatory cytokines + Adhesion markers **Related to ATHEROSCLEROSIS**

2. INFLAMMATORY, NON-ATHEROSCLEROTIC DISEASES

	Disease	Clinical features	Neuroimaging
1.	**HSP/IgA** Henoch–Schönlein Purpura (IgA vasculitis)	Usual onset in childhood Rarely, adult onset • Purpura seen on back and limbs • Abdominal surgery • Arthropathy • Renal disease **In Adults: Association with Adenocarcinoma lung** has been reported	MRI shows: Bilateral infarcts Angiography shows: Areas of stenosis in MCA/ACA
2.	**ABRA** Amyloid beta-related angiitis	Rare complication of cerebral amyloid angiopathy Shares features with primary angiitis of CNS Sub-acute onset (1–2 months) headache Seizures, mental changes, neuro deficits EEG: Generalized Slow waves CSF: Mild lymphocytic (10 cells), **high protein** Rx: Steroids + cyclophosphamide	MRI brain shows: • Lepto **meningeal enhancement** (MC*) • White matter changes • Infarcts • Micro-hemorrhages • Cortical hemosidrin
3.	**CAA** Cerebral amyloid angiopathy	Clinically presents with • TIA (transient ischemic attacks • LOBAR BLEED (**important) • Dementia BOSTON criteria: Used for diagnosis May be associated with superficial siderosis	Deposition of beta amyloid is seen in • Medium-sized vessels • Cortex • Sub-cortex • Leptomeninges

CAA	ABRA	PA-CNS (primary angiitis of CNS)
Figure 1.4 Schematic representation of CAA.	Figure 1.5 Schematic representation of ABRA.	Figure 1.6 Schematic representation of PA-CNS.
Amyloid deposits ++	Amyloid deposits ++ Inflammation ++	Inflammation ++ Vasculitis +

(Continued)

(Continued)

4.	**Temporal arteritis**	Onset >50 years • H/o weight loss, • Blurring of vision • Scalp tenderness + • Temporal artery pulse not palpable • Fundus: Pale disc with edema **Rx: Urgent treatment with steroids needed to save vision**	Temporal Artery Doppler: Increased diameter and hypoechoic wall thickening (halo sign) of the superficial temporal artery MRI with vessel wall imaging can also be done
5.	**Takayasu arteritis**	Onset of disease <40 years Vasculitis involves aorta and its branches • Stenosis, occlusions of large vessels • Dilatations and aneurysms • Renal HTN, CHF, CAD • Claudication of Upper extremities > Lower extremity • Decreased brachial artery pulsations • Blood pressure difference >10 mmHg in two arms • Bruit heard over subclavian or abdominal aorta Rx: High-dose steroids	ACR criteria used for diagnosis (3/6 criteria need to be fulfilled) Gold standard: ANGIOGRAPHY • **Long segment, tapered, smooth** stenosis • Frank occlusions, collateral vessels

3. NON-INFLAMMATORY NON-ATHEROSCLEROTIC DISEASES

1.	Sneddon's syndrome	**Small and medium vessel vasculopathy Neuro-cutaneous vasculopathy Seen in young females** • **Livedo racemose** Dusky erythematous or violaceous **rash with net-like appearance** • Affects limbs >> Trunk/Buttocks/Face • Neurological symptoms: Stroke • Thrombosis of intracranial vessels • HTN and migraine • **Heart: CAD/MI/ Valvular ds/ murmurs** • Endarteritis obliterans in the skin and the kidney • APLA + in 30–50% patients: May suggest overlap Biopsy shows: Intimal **endothelial proliferation** and thrombosis of arterioles and compensatory capillary dilatation	 Figure 1.7 Difference between livedo reticularis and racemose. Livedo reticularis is due to vaso-constriction and is temporary MRI brain: Cortical and sub-cortical watershed infarctions (embolic-like pattern)

2.	Moyamoya disease	Steno-occlusive disease Involves the Terminal ICA Bimodal incidence: 5 years and 45 years Can be Secondary to (Moyamoya syndrome) • NF-1 (neurofibromatosis-1) • PAN (polyarteritis nodosa) • SCA (spino-cerebellar ataxia) • Down syndrome Attacks of cerebral ischemia classically during • Exercise • Hyper-ventilation	Neuroimaging signs in Moyamoya disease • Puff of smoke (abnormal dilated collaterals) • IVY sign on FLAIR • Branches of ECA supply dura and base of skull Rx: Antiplatelets, bypass surgery (ECA-MCA bypass) • No role of anticoagulants
3.	FMD Fibromuscular dysplasia	Onset: Women, childbearing age Involves the medium-sized vessels Can be found in about 15–20% patients with cervical dissections	Angiography findings • Stenosis, occlusions • Cervical arteries + Renal arteries • Cervical artery dissections Renal FMD: Contrast MRA very sensitive for diagnosis
4.	HHT Hereditary hemorrhagic telangiectasia	Autosomal dominant History of: Epistaxis + telangiectasia Telangiectasia seen in: Skin + lips + mucus membranes Ischemic stroke: May be the first presentation Strokes are associated with pulmonary AVM in 30% patients Stroke prevention: Closure of pulmonary AVM	Asymptomatic AVMs seen in • Lung • Liver • Brain and spine
5.	Homocystinuria	Rare autosomal recessive disease Resembles Marfan's syndrome • Marfanoid habitus • Skeletal: Pectus excavatum • Ectopis lentis, myopia • Learning difficulties, developmental delay • But **NO JOINT HYPERMOBILITY** • Thromboembolic events, stroke, CVT	Blood investigations • Macrocytic anemia • Elevated blood and urine homocysteine Genetics: Cystathione beta-synthetase deficiency Rx • B6 supplementation • B12 supplementation • Methionine restricted diet

(Continued)

(Continued)

6.	Fabry disease	X-linked disorder The common clinical features are: • Burning feet, hypo-hidrosis • Abdominal pain, • Post-prandial diarrhea, weight loss • Exercise intolerance • **Severe pain after heat** (stress/illness/fatigue) • HOCM, arrythmia, HTN • SNHL in 50% • Angiokeratomas in 40% Age-wise presentation • In 20s and 30s: Micro-albuminuria, proteinuria • In 40s and 50s: CKD	Cause: Alpha-galactosidase A deficiency The previously mentioned enzyme is seen in: WBC, blood Rx: Enzyme replacement therapy

4. MISCELLANEOUS CEREBROVASCULAR DISEASES

a. CCF: Carotico-cavernous fistula. There are dilated conjunctival vessels, or "corkscrew"-like vessels.

b. SAH: Sub-arachnoid hemorrhage. Guidelines for screening in family members if: >1 first-degree relative (mother/father/siblings) has SAH.

c. Post-cardiac surgery strokes. Hemodynamic stroke in post-cardiac surgery patients are seen in ~40% patients, compared to 2–3% in general population. The pathogenesis is a combination of hypo-perfusion and embolic strokes. Hence, it is better to maintain MAP at 80–100 mmHg rather than 40–50 mmHg.

d. Strokes are more common with aortic procedures than simple CABG.

5. THROMBOLYSIS IN STROKE

Indication for thrombolysis: <4.5 hours from the onset of deficits till the start of thrombolytic agent.

BOX 1.1   RELATIVE CONTRAINDICATIONS

1. >75 years age
2. Hepatic dysfunction
3. Pregnancy
4. Recent trauma
5. Anticoagulant use
6. Recent GIT or GUS bleeding
7. Recent major surgery (OBG delivery, organ biopsy, CABG)
8. DM hemorrhagic retinopathy
9. Recent puncture at non-compressible site
10. Active peptic ulcer

Contraindications: Absolute Contraindications for Thrombolysis in Stroke

a. Any history of ICH (intracerebral hemorrhage).
b. BP >185/100 mmHg.
c. Ischemic stroke in the last 3 months.
d. Known intracranial neoplasm.
e. Known structural lesion (AVM).
f. Active internal bleeding (excluding menses).
g. Suspected aortic dissection or pericarditis.
h. Head trauma or brain surgery in last 6 months.
i. Major surgery, trauma, bleeding in last 3–6 weeks.
j. Special situations
   i. Heparin in last 48 hours.
   ii. INR >1.7.
   iii. Platelets <1lac.
   iv. Seizures at onset.
   v. Bacterial endocarditis.

Complication: Angioedema during Thrombolysis

a. Transient, mild phenomenon.
b. Involves contralateral face.
c. Risk factors: Patient on ACE inhibitors and insula infarction.
d. Insula infarction: Cause sympatho-vagal imbalance—Causes angioedema and arrythmias.
e. Autonomic dysregulation plays a role in angioedema.

6. SPECIFIC NEUROIMAGING SIGNS IN CEREBROVASCULAR DISEASES

a. The *caput medusa*, a cluster of veins resembling a head of snakes, refers to veins draining into a larger collector vein that usually is on the surface of the brain. Seen in **Developmental venous anomalies (venous angiomas) of the brain, where a number of veins drain centrally towards a single vein**. The appearance is reminiscent of Medusa, a gorgon of Greek mythology, who was defeated by Perseus.
b. The *ivy sign* refers to the MRI appearance of patients with Moyamoya disease or Moyamoya syndrome. Prominent leptomeningeal collaterals: On FLAIR images were defined as **linear high signal intensity** along the cortical sulci (sulcal hyperintensities) or brain surface in the cerebral hemisphere. Diffuse leptomeningeal enhancement resembles creeping ivy on stones. DSA would show puff of smoke appearance in Moya Moya disease.
c. *Puff of smoke* sign describes the characteristic angiographic appearance of **tiny abnormal intracranial collateral vessel networks** in Moyamoya disease. Moyamoya disease is a non-atherosclerotic steno-occlusive disease affecting bilateral distal (terminal) ICA.
d. Bilateral thalamic paramedian infarction: Seen in 0.1–2% of all strokes. Etiology is usually, cardioembolic. Causes include occlusion of
   i. Artery of Percheron (single dominant thalamo-perforator).
   ii. Basilar top occlusion.
   iii. VOG (vein of Galen) or **straight sinus CVT**. Thalamus is drained via perforating veins into the INTERNAL cerebral vein and BASAL veins. The ICV and BV join to form the great cerebral VOG. **VOG then joins ISS (inferior sagittal sinus) to form the SS (straight sinus)**.

7. NICE GUIDELINES IN STROKE

Recognition	TIA/Stroke	Outside the hospital: Use FAST (Face, Arm, Speech, Time) Inside the hospital: Use ROSIER tool
	Immediately (in the ER)	Exclude hypoglycemia (check blood sugars) Give aspirin 300 mg stat
TIA (Transient Ischemic Attack)		
Refer the patient		To TIA clinic within 24 hours
		No need to use ABCD2 score
Secondary prevention		Another agent for secondary prevention is added to aspirin As soon as diagnosis of TIA made
Brain imaging	CT brain	Do not do CT unless any alternative diagnosis to be excluded
	MRI brain	MRI has to be done after specialist assessment to see the territory of stroke And rule out bleed To be done on the same day
Carotid	Imaging	Everyone who is a candidate for CEA should have carotid imaging
	Urgent CEA (carotid-end-arterectomy)	NASCET 50–99% with acute non-disabling stroke or TIA Refer urgently to specialist center, to be done within 1 week Receive best medical management
		  Figure 1.8 Carotid artery stenosis grade.
	NSCET <50% ESCT <70%	No surgery Best medical management only: Diet, lifestyle changes, BP management, cholesterol management, antiplatelet drugs
STROKE		
CT scan urgently indicated	Non-contrast CT if	a. Patient has an indication for thrombolysis b. Patient is on anticoagulants c. Patient has a known bleeding tendency d. Low GCS <13 e. Unexplained progression or fluctuation of deficits f. Presence of papilledema, neck stiffness, fever g. Severe headache at onset
CT angiography if		h. Thrombectomy indicated
CT or MR perfusion if		i. Patient presents in extended window (if >6 hours)

	Perform within 24 hours	A CT scan of the brain can be performed within 24 hours in everyone if urgent not indicated
Alteplase	Administer	Alteplase has to be administered within 4.5 hours

	Settings	Alteplase can only be administered in:
		• Stroke units
		• ER with trained staff
		  • Nursing staff trained to give level 1 and level 2 care
		  • Immediate access to imaging and staff trained in interpreting

Mechanical thrombectomy	<6 hours	Class I indicated in patients presenting in <6 hours with anterior circulation LVO (large vessel occlusion)
	6–24 hours/wake up stroke	Mechanical thrombectomy in extended window performed only if: • CT perfusion shows perfusion deficits or • MRI brain shows diffusion-FLAIR mismatch Both these indicate a limited core and significant area to salvage
		Pre-**functional mRS <3, NIHSS >5**
Secondary prevention		
Any Ischemic stroke/ TIA	Aspirin 300 mg	Start immediately or within 24 hours, after bleed is excluded
	Aspirin rectal or Ryles tube	If they have dysphagia
	Aspirin 300 mg	**Given for x 14 days**
	PPI	If dyspepsia with aspirin
	Alternate drugs if	Hypersensitivity to aspirin Severe dyspepsia to low-dose aspirin
ICA Dissection		Aspirin or anticoagulants
CVT		Heparin followed by warfarin (INR 2–3)
APLA		Same as any AIS
Atrial fibrillation	Disabling stroke	**Aspirin 300 mg x 14 days** Then start anticoagulation
Prosthetic valve	Disabling stroke	**Aspirin 300 mg x 7 days** Then start anticoagulation
Proximal DVT/PE	+ stroke If hemorrhagic stroke	Anticoagulation Anticoagulation or DVT filters
ICH with warfarin		Immediate PCC and iv vitamin K
STATINS		
	Acute ischemic stroke	Immediate statins not indicated in AIS
	Already taking statin	If a patient of stroke is already taking statins, they can continue taking them
ICU management		
Oxygen	Supplementation	Only if saturation <95%
Sugars		Maintain 4–11 mmol/L
BP (ICH)	Immediate lowering if	<6 hours onset with SBP 150–220 mmHg
BP (ICH)	Immediate lowering if	>6 hours onset with SBP >220 mmHg
	Target	<140 mmHg; drop 60 mmHg per hour

(*Continued*)

(Continued)

ICU management (Contd)		
	Do not lower if	GCS <6 Going to have decompression Massive hematoma, poor prognosis Structural lesions: AVM, aneurysm, neoplasm
BP (AIS)	Thrombolysis	<185/100 mmHg
	>4.5 hours	Only if there is HTN emergency with • HTN nephropathy • HTN encephalopathy • HTN CHF/MI • Dissection • Eclampsia

ICU management: Surgery in ICH is indicated if neuroimaging shows hydrocephalus**		
	Rarely require surgery if	Following situations rarely require surgery • Small deep hemorrhage • Lobar hemorrhage w/o hydrocephalus • Large hemorrhage but significant comorbidities • Posterior fossa hemorrhage • GCS <8, unless due to hydrocephalus

ICU management: Decompressive surgery in ischemic stroke if		
	Decompression done within 48 hours**	MCA infarct with NIHSS >15 Decreased LOC with a score of 1 or more on NIHSS que 1a CT infarction >**50% of MCA** territory; MRI diffusion **infarction >145 cm³** Discuss the risks, benefits, outcomes and prognosis with family members

ICU management: Nutrition		
	Within 24 hours**	Screen swallowing by trained HCW before giving food, fluid or meds
	Within 24 hours, but not later than 72 hours	If basic screening has some problems: • Ensure specialist evaluation
	Instrument examination if	? Aspiration Need tube feeding for 3 days
	Tube feeding	RT within 24 hours If RT not tolerated—gastrostomy or nasal birdle tube

Nutrition		
		Screen all AIS for malnutrition at admission And every week for in patients Use MUST scoring Use BMI, unintentional body loss %Supplements only for patients who are at risk of malnutrition

Early mobilization		
		Out of bed as soon as possible (within **24 hours—AVERT trial**) If they need help to sit/stand or walk, do not offer High-intensity mobilization within 24 hours (from AVERT trial)
3 additional out-of-bed sessions compared with usual care Focuses on sitting, standing and walking (that is, out of bed) activity		

8. RISK STRATIFICATION SCORES IN STROKE

a. **ROSIER** tool: ER assessment.

b. NIHSS: National Institute of Heath Stroke Score—A 1-point increase in NIHSS reduces chances of good outcome by 17%.
   - NIHSS 1–4: Minor stroke.
   - NIHSS 5–15: Moderate.
   - NIHSS 16–20: Moderate to severe.
   - NIHSS >20: Severe stroke.

c. **CHADS^{2}VASc score** and adjusted annual stroke risk from AF: (CHF = LVEF <40%).
   - 0 = 0
   - 1 = 1.3%
   - 2 = 2.2%
   - 3 = 3.2%
   - 4 = 4%
   - 5 = 6.7%
   - 6 = 9.9%
   - 7 = 9.6%
   - 8 = 6.7%
   - 9 = 15%

d. **HASBLED** score and risk of bleed per 100-patient years.
   - 0 = 1.13
   - 1 = 1.01
   - 2 = 1.88
   - 3 = 3.74
   - 4 = 12.5

EPILEPSY AND SLEEP DISORDERS

1. ILAE DEFINITION OF EPILEPSY

ILAE: International League Against Epilepsy

A person is labelled to have epilepsy if they have:	
2 or more unprovoked or reflex seizures	Occurring 24 hours apart
1 unprovoked or reflex seizure +	Probability of recurrence 60% in 10 years
Diagnosis of Epilepsy syndrome	Abnormal EEG
An unprovoked seizure +	Abnormal MRI brain

- Seizure + EEG abnormal = 2 times the risk of recurrence compared to seizure + normal EEG

2. IDIOPATHIC GENERALIZED EPILEPSY (IGE)

a. IGE = Idiopathic generalized epilepsy. IGE includes
  i. CAE (childhood absence epilepsy).
  ii. JME (juvenile myoclonic epilepsy).
  iii. JAE (juvenile absence epilepsy).
  iv. GTCS (generalized tonic clonic seizures).
b. All patients having new-onset seizures should have MRI brain, except those with a diagnosis of IGE or childhood self-limiting focal epilepsy.

3. TRAVEL REGULATIONS FOR PATIENTS WITH EPILEPSY

Air Travel

- Air travel (flight): Can travel 24 hours after a seizure otherwise they need medical clearance for travel within 24 hours of seizure.

Car Drive

Clinical condition	Cannot drive for
Awake seizures	12 months
Seizure when asleep	1 year
1st seizure with Loss of Consciousness (when awake)	6 months
1st seizure with abnormal EEG or MRI abnormal	1 year
Repeat seizure when AED stopped/reduced	6 months on AED and no seizure
Seizure when asleep + awake	3 years + seizure allowed in sleep

DOI: 10.1201/b23306-2

Bus/Lorry Drive

- One-off seizure: No AED required and no seizure for 5 years.
- >1 seizure: No AED required and no seizure for 10 years + >2% risk of another seizure.

4. AUTOIMMUNE CAUSES OF EPILEPSY

    a. Causes of NORSE (New-Onset Refractory Status Epilepticus).
- i. 50% cryptogenic.
- ii. 40% autoimmune and paraneoplastic (Most common: NMDA encephalitis).
- iii. Infectious causes: (EBV, CMV, VZV, mycoplasma, syphilis).
- iv. Leptomeningeal carcinomatosis.

5. PEDIATRIC SEIZURES

a.	Most common cause of neonatal seizures: HIE (hypoxic ischemic encephalopathy) = 30–40% Most common cause of pediatric NORSE: Infections	
b.	Febrile seizure (FS)	Risk of further epilepsy in a patient with FS if <ul><li>Focal onset</li><li>Duration >15 minutes</li><li>Multiple seizures lasting >24 hours</li><li>Family history of epilepsy</li></ul>

6. PEDIATRIC EPILEPSY SYNDROMES

		Clinical	Investigations and treatment
1.	GAMT deficiency: Treatable epilepsy	GAMT = Guanidinoacetate Methyl Transferase Autosomal recessive disorder Clinical features:<ul><li>Developmental delay</li><li>Learning difficulty, AUTISM</li><li>Behavior abnormalities</li><li>**SPEECH severely** affected</li></ul>Seizure types: GTCS, atypical absence, drop attack	**LOW serum CREATININE**** MRI: Bilateral globus pallidus changes MRS: Depleted creatinine in brain Genetic testing from blood or saliva Rx: Supplement creatine Late Rx also improves seizure control
2.	Dravet SMEI: Severe myoclonic epilepsy of infancy	Refractory epilepsy in infancy Clinical presentation:<ul><li>Febrile convulsive Status f/b</li><li>Non-febrile clonic UL seizures</li><li>Long duration and frequent seizures</li><li>Family h/o febrile seizures +</li><li>Regression of milestones +</li></ul>**DO NOT give**: PHT, CBZ, LTG, VBT	EEG: Multifocal and generalized spikes **Photosensitivity seen** in 40% **SCN1A** mutation in 75% Rx: VPA, topiramate, Clobazam. Newer drugs: Stiripentol, Fenfluramine*
3.	West syndrome	Infantile spasms	Vigabatrine used as monotherapy
4.	LKS Landau–Kleffner syndrome	Onset 2–10 years (mostly 5–7 years) Clinical features:<ul><li>Verbal auditory agnosia</li><li>Fails to understand meaning of sounds</li><li>Reduction in spontaneous speech</li></ul>	EEG: Spike and wave discharges in posterior temporal/temporo-parietal, temporo-occipital areas bilaterally Recovery of language is variable

		Clinical	Investigations and treatment
5.	Myoclonic–atonic epilepsy (Doose syndrome)	Onset 6 months–6 years Starts with GTCS; later on falls (atonic seizure), myoclonic and absence seizures are also seen	Try ketogenic diet early in Rx (before 2nd or 3rd AED)
6.	JME Juvenile myoclonic epilepsy	Mainly in adolescent age group Early morning GTCS Occasional myoclonic jerks	Lamotrigine can aggravate myoclonic jerk In pregnant women: Use Levetiracetam
7.	Rasmussen's encephalitis	Childhood-onset focal seizures Initially seizures are less frequent Then there is an acute phase with progressive hemi-atrophy, hemiparesis Hemianopia, cognitive decline	Serum: GluR3 Antibodies + MRI: Hemiatrophy brain Rx: IVIG in early stages of disease Hemispherectomy in late stages (for seizure control)
8.	Sunflower syndrome	Self-induced photosensitive epilepsy Seizures induced by: Waving hand across vision while staring at sun Onset: Females of age 6–8 years Seizure type: Eyelid myoclonia With or without absence	EEG: Generalized spike and wave discharges (GSWD) Photoparoxysmal response++ Rx: VPA (valproate) LEV (levetiracetam) and LTG (Lamotrigine) in adolescents
9.	Jeavons syndrome	Similar to sunflower syndrome But seizures are stimulated by closing eyes	Also called epilepsy with eyelid myoclonia
10.	Gray matter heterotopia	Multiple seizures	Imaging types <ul><li>Sub-ependymal (peri-ventricular)</li><li>Sub-cortical</li><li>Band heterotopia</li></ul>
11.	CAE Childhood absence epilepsy	Clinically, school-going child with staring episodes lasting few seconds Child appears to have gone blank May have convulsions GTCS	EEG: 3–4 Hz slow spike and wave discharges May be anterior dominant Seizure precipitated by Hyperventilation Rx: Ethosuximide preferred > VPA Ethosuximide is less effective if GTCS
12.	GRIIN 2a mutation	Atypical childhood epilepsy with Centro-temporal spikes Seizure type: Facial twitching + and – myoclonus Atypical absence Drop attacks	EEG: Mildly slow background Centro-temporal spikes (CTS) arising independently from both hemispheres
13.	CHRN a2	Sleep hypermotor activity	
14.	SLC2a1	Conditions associated with GLUT deficiency Myoclonic atonic epilepsy	

(*Continued*)

(Continued)

		Clinical	Investigations and treatment
15.	KCNQ2	Self-limiting infantile epilepsy	
16.	NFLE Nocturnal frontal lobe epilepsy	Onset in puberty or adulthood Family history + Multiple episodes of seizures Seizure type: Suddenly raises arms in sleep Stereotyped behavior: Vocalization, Frightened expression, fear Complex movements Moves around Dances/chorea/ballismus/pedalling-type movements seen	EEG: Frontal lobe onset seizures FLEP score used to differentiate frontal lobe seizures from non-epileptic and psychogenic events

7. NON-EPILEPTIC SYNDROMES

		Clinical	Investigations and diagnosis
1.	POTS Postural tachycardia syndrome	Transient LOC (loss of consciousness) while standing Low blood pressure and tachycardia	Tilt table test Presence of autonomic neuropathy/Diabetes mellitus
2.	PNES Non-epileptic syndrome	Long duration of seizures (>5–10 minutes) Asynchronous jerking Pelvic thrusting Back arching Closed eyes	EEG will be normal Provocative tests positive

8. MESS TRIAL—RECURRENCE

a. The MRC Multicentre Trial for Early Epilepsy and Single Seizures predicted the risk of recurrence of seizure after a single seizure.

   i. *Low risk*: Prognostic index 0: Single seizure + normal EEG + no neurological disease.

   ii. *Medium risk*: Prognostic index 1: 2–3 seizures + normal EEG, no neurological disease.

   iii. *High risk*: Prognostic index 2–3: >4 seizures or abnormal EEG/neurological disease +.

Risk	Treatment	Probability of seizure at 1 year	Probability of seizure at 3 years	Probability of seizure at 5 years
Low	Start	0.26	0.35	0.39
	Delay	0.19	0.28	0.30
Medium	Start	0.24	0.35	0.39
	Delay	0.35	0.50	0.56
High	Start	0.36	0.46	0.50
	Delay	0.59	0.67	0.73

Kim LG. Johnson TL. Marson AG et al. Prediction of risk of seizure recurrence after a single seizure and early epilepsy: further results from the MESS trial. Lancet Neurol 2006;5:317–322

Figure 2.1 (Courtesy of Elsevier).

9. LOCALIZATION-RELATED EPILEPSY (LRE)

	Seizure semiology	Localization/Etiology
1.	Fear expression followed by screaming, agitation f/b kicking: Lasts 10–15 seconds	Ventral/Ventro-medial prefrontal cortex
2.	Subjective feeling of fear	Temporal lobe seizures
3.	Uncontrolled laughter: Gelastic seizures	Hypothalamic hamartoma
4.	Déjà vu cognitive seizures	Left temporal localization
5.	Hyperphagia	Kleine-Levine syndrome
6.	Impaired verbal memory	After left cerebral resection

10. SPECIAL INVESTIGATIONS IN EPILEPSY

a. Indications for intracranial EEG recording.
   i. Proximity of the seizure-onset zone to eloquent cortex.
   ii. Lesions with poorly defined borders.
   iii. Multiple lesions.
   iv. Discordant test results or another source of uncertainty about the seizure-onset zone.
   v. Prior history of surgical failure.

11. DRUG TREATMENT OF EPILSEPSY

a. For focal-onset seizures: Phenytoin, CBZ, oxcarbazepine.
b. For GTCS: Valproate is the best.
c. GTCS adjunctive Rx: Levetiracetam, Topiramate, Lamotrigine, Perampanel.
d. Cenobamate: Newer drug which is sodium channel blocker and enhances GABA.
e. Cannabidiol increases the concentration of N-desmethylclobazam, which can result in somnolence.

12. STIMULATION TREATMENT FOR EPILEPSY

a. VNS: Vagal nerve stimulation
   i. Used for multiple different focus.
   ii. Cannot do resection or Response neurostimulation.
b. Response neurostimulation: Used when
   i. Close to eloquent cortex—cannot resect.

13. SPECIFIC SIDE EFFECTS RELATED TO ANTIEPILEPTIC DRUGS (AEDs)

a. Vigabatrin: Visual peripheral loss.
b. Combined oral contraceptive pills reduce AED levels by 40–60%.
   i. **LTG levels reduced >>> VPA.**
c. CBZ: Enzyme inducer—Reduces level of progestins.
d. Topiramate: Acute **glaucoma: Occurs within 2 weeks** painful red eye. Diagnosed if 3 or more of
   i. IOP >21.
   ii. Conjunctival injection.
   iii. Corneal edema.
   iv. Mid-dilated non-reactive pupil.
   v. Shallow anterior chamber.
e. VPA (valproate) is contraindicated in MELAS/mitochondrial diseases because
   i. VPA interferes with respiratory chain.
f. Mitochondrial disease/epilepsy: Can try LTG, LEV, GBP, Zonisamide.
g. VPA (Valproate): Causes acute pancreatitis.

14. SEIZURES AND PSYCHIATRY

a. Psychiatric side effects seen in
  i. LEV (levetiracetam).
  ii. AMPA modulators–perampanel.
  iii. Phenobarbitone.
  iv. Zonisamide.
  v. Pregabalin.
b. Lowest psychiatric side effects seen with sodium channel blockers: CBZ.
c. Rx of psychiatric side effects
  i. Risperidone.
  ii. Olanzapine.
  iii. Quetiapine.
d. ADHD + seizures: Use stimulant + AED—Major improvement in concentration by 60–80%.

15. SYMPTOMATIC OR PROVOKED SEIZURES

a. Acute post-seizure epilepsy: Seizures within 7 days of stroke.
b. Most common cause of focal seizure in elderly = stroke.
c. Brain tumours: Low-grade brain tumours can cause seizures.
d. Seizures in glioneural tumours: More common in DNET (100%) >> ganglioglioma
  i. Occur in childhood.
  ii. Common in temporal lobes.
  iii. MRI: Multicystic lesions.
  iv. Lack mass effect.
  v. Do not enhance, T2 hyperintense.

16. RISK OF PSYCHOSIS IN EPILEPSY IF

a. Early age at onset of seizures.
b. Febrile seizures or febrile Status epilepticus.
c. Presence of structural brain lesion.
d. MRI: Left temporal focus, Hippocampal sclerosis.
e. Family h/o psychosis.
f. Poorly controlled seizures on AED.
g. Risk of psychiatric side effects less with sodium channel blockers.

17. RISK OF SUDEP (SUDDEN UNEXPLAINED DEATH IN EPILEPSY) IF

a. Young age patients: 15–20 years.
b. Seizures associated with learning difficulties.
c. Poorly controlled seizures: >15 seizures per month.
d. Patient taking >2 AEDS.

18. UK ECLAMPSIA TRIAL DEFINITIONS

Eclampsia Definition

a. Seizures in pregnancy or within 10 days of delivery with 2 of these (in 24 hours)
  i. Hypertension (DBP >90 mmHg, or increase of >25 mmHg).
  ii. Proteinuria 1+ or 0.3 g/24 hours.
  iii. Thrombocytopenia <1 lac.
  iv. AST levels >42.
b. The drug of choice in eclampsia is magnesium sulfate—it causes cerebral vasodilatation.

c. Urgent delivery indicated if
   i. Progressive headache.
   ii. Scotoma, blurring of vision present.
   iii. Epigastric pain.
   iv. DBP >110 mmHg.
   v. Coagulopathy.
   vi. High creatinine or liver enzymes.
   vii. Clonus.
d. Maintain BP >130/80 mmHg for placental perfusion.
e. Immediately reduce BP if >170/110 mmHg.

19. SPECIFIC OR DIAGNOSTIC EEG AND MRI FINDINGS IN EPILEPSY

a. EEG potentials are produced due to
   i. Post-synaptic potentials in apical dendrites.
   ii. Of layer IV and V pyramidal cells.
b. Essential MRI sequences to be done in epilepsy.
   i. T1.
   ii. FLAIR.
   iii. Coronal T2.
   iv. Contrast T1 and SWI (susceptibility) are optional sequences.

	Syndrome	EEG findings	Other specific/Diagnostic points
1.	LGS (Lennox–Gastaut syndrome)	Diffuse slow background Multifocal spikes or Slow spike and wave discharges with • Bursts of generalized fast activity	Childhood onset Multiple seizure types Cognitive decline
2.	CAE (Childhood absence epilepsy)	3–4 Hz slow spike and wave discharges May be anterior dominant Seizure precipitated by Hyperventilation ++	School-going child with Staring episodes Ethosuximide > VPA Ethosuximide less effective if GTCS
3.	Anti-NMDA-encephalitis	EEG: Extreme delta brush pattern (EDB) Or generalized rhythmic delta activity (GRDA) EDB means: Slow delta activity superimposed on 1–2-second bursts of low amplitude high frequency	Most common cause of NORSE • Clinically autonomic features ++ predominate the clinical features
4.	Anti-LG1-encephalitis	EEG: Temporal epileptiform discharges or frontal slow activity Types of seizures • Dyscognitive • Gelastic • Autonomic	Facio-brachial dystonic seizures (FBDS) MRI: Hippocampal intensities (mesial temporal) Hyponatremia
5.	Anti-DPPX encephalitris	EEG: Non-specific slowing may be seen	Clinically—GIT manifestations: • Diarrhea very common • CNS hyperexcitability • Hyperekplexia, myoclonus
6.	GFAP disease		MRI in GFAP astrocytopathy: Diffuse perivascular enhancement radiating out from the lateral ventricles

20. WWE (WOMEN WITH EPILEPSY)

a. In first-ever prospective obstetric trial in patients with epilepsy: There was no difference in fertility parameters like time to pregnancy.
b. Clobazam, oxcarbazepine and rufinamide decrease both ethinylestradiol and progestins.
c. Perampanel decreases just progestins (*P reduces P*).
d. Zonisamide—no effect on OCP.
e. In pregnancy: 15–20% women complain of worsening of seizure control.

DISORDERS OF CRANIAL NERVES AND VISUAL SYSTEM

Abbreviations

- *CISS MRI*: Constructive interference in steady state MRI
- *PAN*: Polyarteritis nodosa
- *SCA*: Superior cerebellar artery
- *SLE*: Systemic lupus erythematosus
- *SOF*: Superior orbital fissure
- *TN*: Trigeminal neuralgia
- *V1, V2, V3*: Ophthalmic, maxillary and mandibular divisions of trigeminal nerve

1. DISORDERS OF THE VISUAL SYSTEM CRANIAL NERVES

	Disease	Clinical features	Diagnosis and treatment
1.	SOF syndrome v/s Orbital apex syndrome	Both these syndromes will involve • III, IV, VI cranial nerves • V1 and V2 cranial nerves But orbital apex syndrome will also involve the optic nerve • Orbital apex = SOF + optic nerve	MRI brain shows: Vasogenic edema • In sub-cortical or rarely cortical • bilateral parieto-occipital regions
		Posterior cavernous syndrome = Orbital apex + Maxillary V2 division + Oculo-sympathetic fibre involvement	

2. DISORDERS OF THE TRIGEMINAL NERVE

	Disease	Clinical features	Diagnosis and treatment
1.	TN Trigeminal neuralgia	Sudden Sharp or shooting or lancinating Short lasting Severe pain Sudden bouts of pain Lasts for a very short time Triggered by common daily activities: • Brushing • Shaving • Chewing • Speaking • Combing	MRI brain may be normal. To demonstrate a vascular cause (loop of artery), we can do a gradient echo (CISS-3d MRI) Cause of trigeminal neuralgia • 75% due to SCA loop • Tortuous basilar artery • Trigemino cerebellar artery • Persistent trigeminal artery

(Continued)

DOI: 10.1201/b23306-3

(Continued)

	Disease	Clinical features	Diagnosis and treatment
2.	TTS Trigeminal trophic syndrome	Complication of sensory loss in the distribution of the trigeminal nerve Pathophysiology: Either due to central or peripheral cause Etiology: Herpes zoster, lateral medullary syndrome, trauma, syphilis Clinically: Painless ulcerations • Can occur weeks to years later • Induced by severe paresthesia	Rx: Avoid trauma Can use: • Neuropathic pain drugs like Gabapentin, amitriptyline

3. DISORDERS OF THE FACIAL NERVE

	Disease	Clinical features	Diagnosis and treatment
1.	Bell's palsy	The classical LMN type of facial nerve palsy Cause: Idiopathic • Bells palsy term is labelled when there is no apparent cause for LMN facial palsy Clinically • Weakness of one half of the face • Involves forehead and eye closure muscles • Bell's phenomenon + Recurrence seen in: **7% in 10** years	Excellent prognosis Rx: Steroids • 1 mg/kg or 60 mg x 5 days, then rapid taper • Usual duration of therapy 8–10 days Steroids have been shown to be superior to placebo for treatment of Bell's palsy Addition of acyclovir has not been shown to be superior to placebo
2.	Ramsay Hunt syndrome/ Herpes zoster oticus	Shingles affecting the facial nerve near the ear Ear pain Hearing loss May also have LMN facial palsy	Acyclovir/Antivirals recommended for treatment
3.	Melkersson– Rosenthal syndrome	Triad of • Recurrent orofacial/lip edema • Fissured tongue • LMN facial palsy The most common presentation is recurrent orofacial/lip edema May have a mono-symptomatic or recurrent course	Biopsy: Non-caseating granuloma Rx: Steroids Edema of facial palsy Remits early but can recur and can become permanent Figure 3.1 A patient of Melkersson–Rosenthal syndrome.

4. DISORDERS OF THE LOWER CRANIAL NERVES

	Disease	Clinical features	Diagnosis and treatment
1.	Numb chin syndrome	Sensory neuropathy syndrome Clinically presents with numbness in the lower lips, chin and jaw In the distribution of terminal branch of mandibular nerve (V3) Causes • Breast and prostate cancer • Dental procedures • Diabetes neuropathy • Sarcoidosis, SLE • Sjogren's syndrome • PAN • Infections: Lyme disease • HIV-AIDS	In the presence of malignancy, numb chin syndrome signifies a poor prognosis Average survival = **7 months** Figure 3.2 Schematic diagram of distribution of numbness.
2.	Tapia syndrome	Rare disease Characterized by simultaneous unilateral hypoglossal palsy and recurrent laryngeal nerve palsy Cause: Airway injury • Usually follows oro-tracheal intubation • Direct compression and stretching of: Hypoglossal/rec laryngeal nerves Clinically • Dysarthria + dysphonia + swallowing • Recover in few months	 Figure 3.3 A patient with Tapia syndrome.
3.	Radiation neuropathy	Occurs 1–14 years after radiotherapy for cranial tumours like • Pituitary • Chiasmal neoplasms • Ocular neoplasms • Meningioma Most common involvement: Ophthalmic nerve** Site of involvement: Posterior portion/ chiasma** 2nd most common involvement: Hypoglossal nerve palsy	Large doses of radiation pose risk to following structures • >50 Gy to nerve plexus • >60 Gy to cranial nerves • >2.5 Gy per dose pose a high risk

5. NEURO-OPHTHALMOLOGY

Anisocoria

	Testing	Drops
Normal anisocoria	Greater in DARK	1% apraclonidine
Pharmacological anisocoria	Greater in LIGHT No reaction to light No reaction to accommodation	1% Pilocarpine 0.1% Pilocarpine
	Everything is -ve (negative/no reaction) in pharmacologically dilated pupils (anisocoria)	
Oculomotor **p**alsy	Similar to pharmacological but	Reacts to **p**ilocarpine**

(Continued)

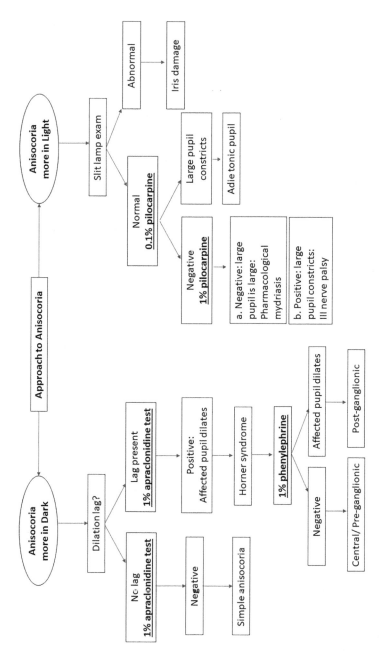

Figure 3.4 Approach to anisocoria.

(Continued)

	Testing	Drops
Adie tonic pupil	Similar to pharmacological but	Reacts to 0.125% dilute pilocarpine**
Horner's syndrome	DARK + dilation lag	
ARP	Light-near dissociation Reacts to near target (within reading range)	

- a. Causes of **pharmacological dilated (pan -ve) pupil**
  - i. Sympathomimetic and parasympatholytic drugs.
  - ii. Adrenaline.
  - iii. Phenylephrine.
  - iv. Apra-clonidine.
  - v. Atropine, Tropicaminde.
  - vi. Scopolamine, ipratropium.

Horner's Syndrome

- a. DARK (Anisocoria is more in dark).
- b. Dilation lag present (pupil dilates after 10–15 seconds in dark; then the difference is less obvious).
- c. Horner pupils shows a very good reaction to cocaine.
- d. It also shows a good reaction to apra-clonidine.
- e. Anisocoria >**0.8 mm after 10% cocaine****: Highly specific for Horner's syndrome.
- f. Apraclonidine: Dilates Horner pupil, constricts a normal pupil.
- g. How to differentiate which order Horner's.
  - i. Hydroxy-amphetamine dilates 1st- and 2nd-order Horner's.
  - ii. Phenylephrine dilates only 3rd post-ganglionic Horner's.

Causes of different types of Horner's syndrome	
1st-order Horner's	Brainstem lesions C-spine lesions C8–T2 spine lesions
2nd-order Horner's	C8–T2 nerve roots Cervical rib Lower brachial plexus injury Lung apex tumours Subclavian artery aneurysm Sympathetic chain
3rd-order Horner's	Carotid artery diseases Aneurysms, dissection Cavernous sinus lesions Base of skull fracture, tumour Herpes zoster

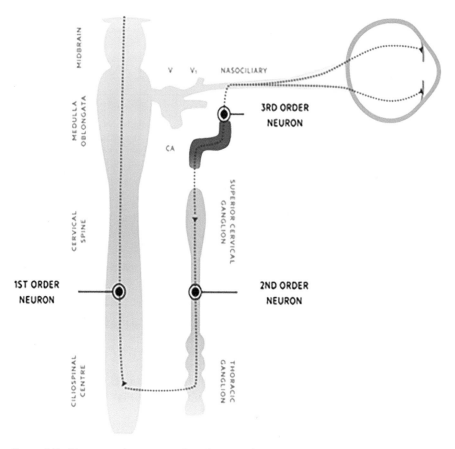

Figure 3.5   Diagrammatic representation of causes of Horner's syndrome.

6. SPECIFIC SYNDROMES IN NEURO-OPHTHALMOLOGY

	Disease	Clinical presentation	Cause, diagnosis and treatment
1.	ARP Argyll Robertson pupil	Light-near dissociation Absent pupillary reflex Preserved accommodation reflex Usually associated with • Vertical upgaze palsy • Supranuclear palsy • Conversion-retraction nystagmus • Collier sign (pathological lid retraction) May affect upgaze alone or Both up and downgaze may be affected	Dorsal midbrain involvement (Parinaud syndrome) Stroke Tumour Brain abscess Demyelination Obstructive hydrocephalus below aqueduct
2.	INO Inter-nuclear ophthalmoplegia	Diplopia Ipsilateral eye does not aDDuct Contralateral eye has aBDuction nystagmus	**MLF lesion (medial longitudinal fasciculus)** (Remember the same side MLF does not duct) So left MLF lesion will cause left INO

	Disease	Clinical presentation	Cause, diagnosis and treatment
3.	One-and-a-half syndrome	INO + horizontal gaze palsy One eye cannot move at all and the other eye only moves outward	**MLF + PPRF lesion** PPRF—parapontine reticular formation Causes • Pontine lesions, hemorrhage • Pontine ischemia • Pontine tumours • Multiple sclerosis • Brainstem infections, tuberculosis
4.	Eight-and-a-half syndrome	One-and-a-half syndrome + 7th nerve palsy	Lesion involving the • Ipsilateral MLF • Ipsilateral VI nerve nucleus • Ipsilateral VII nerve nucleus **Dorsal pons**: Lower pons tegmentum Causes similar to one-and-a-half syndrome
5.	WEBINO Wall-eyed INO Bilateral INO	Not able to aDDuct both eyes ABDuction normal in both eyes ABDuction nystagmus ++ Large-angle esotropia in primary gaze	**Due to brainstem demyelination** Multiple sclerosis
6.	III nerve lesions	Unilateral external ophthalmoplegia Only movement possible is outwards • Ptosis (LPS function) • Pupillary reaction may be abnormal • Eye is down and out	Pupil-sparing III palsy = Diabetes (microvascular damage) Painful and pupil involving III palsy = aneurysms (posterior communicating artery aneurysm)
7.	Superior Oblique (SO) palsy	Vertical diplopia **Bielschowsky test** is used to decide which muscle is paralyzed in cases of hypermetropia **Most cases of SO palsy are congenital due to lax tendon**	Head tilt to opposite side helps to relieve diplopia in SO palsy Right SO palsy = left head tilt Left SO palsy = right head tilt • Helps to relieve diplopia

		Congenital SO palsy
		• 3/4 cases of SO palsy—are congenital
		• Patients will have
		  • Chronic head tilt to opposite side
		  • Facial asymmetry
		  • Face turning to opposite side
		  • Chin depressed
		
		Bielschowsky head tilt is used to decide which muscle is paralyzed
			
			Figure 3.6 Right head tilt in a patient with left SO palsy.

(Continued)

(Continued)

	Disease	Clinical presentation	Cause, diagnosis and treatment
8.	Horizontal diplopia	Depending on the clinical features, we can decide which muscle is paralyzed • Diplopia more in near vision: **MR** • Diplopia more in distant vision: **LR** **MR (medial rectus palsy):** • More while looking to the opposite side LR (lateral rectus palsy) diplopia more in extreme gaze (lateral gaze)	

7. INFECTIOUS DISEASES INVOLVING THE NERVOUS SYSTEM AND EYE

	Disease	Clinical presentation	Cause, diagnosis and management
1.	HsCJD Creutzfeldt–Jakob disease	Heidenhain variant of CJD Isolated **visual symptoms may be seen in early** stages • Visual acuity changes • Visual neglect • Cortical blindness • Palinopsia • Dyschromatopsia • Metamorphopsia • Hallucinations • Cortical blindness These may be followed by cortical symptoms—cognitive decline, ataxia, myoclonus	MRI-DWI (diffusion-weighted imaging): Shows cortical ribboning: Most sensitive early in disease Figure 3.7 Neuroimaging findings in CJD.
2.	THS Tolosa–Hunt syndrome	Severe unilateral periorbital pain with painful recurrent ophthalmoplegia Severe pain Unilateral orbital pain + Ptosis III/IV/VI cranial nerve palsy Relative afferent pupillary defect	Cause: Granulomatous infiltration of cavernous sinus, Superior orbital fissure (SOF) or orbit CSF analysis: Normal MRI brain and orbit: Soft tissue mass seen in cavernous sinus which is • T1 isointense with • Avid Gadolinium enhancement Rx: Exquisitely responsive to steroids—responds within 48 hours

8. INFLAMMATORY DISEASES INVOLVING THE EYE

	Disease	Clinical presentation	Cause, diagnosis and treatment
1.	ON Optic neuritis	Swelling or inflammation of the optic nerve leading to decreased visual acuity • Painless condition • Reduced colour vision The significance of optic neuritis in Neurology is in the fact that it is frequently associated with demyelinating disorders like MS (multiple sclerosis)	

	Disease	Clinical presentation	Cause, diagnosis and treatment
		Unilateral ON—more common with MS Bilateral ON—more common with NMO spectrum disorders, MOGAD As per the ONTT trial (optic neuritis treatment trial): see next table • Cumulative probability of developing MS by 15 years: 50% • If no brain lesion, risk is 25% • If brain lesions present, risk is 75% • Maximum risk is in 5 years • Reduces after 10 years	

Time interval	Cumulative risk	If no brain lesion	If brain lesions are seen
0–5 years	29%	16%	42%
6–10 years	17%	9%	30%
10–15 years	14%	2%	32%

	Disease	Clinical presentation	Cause, diagnosis and treatment
2.	CRION Chronic relapsing inflamma-tory ON	Recurrent ON Patients have pain @ onset May be unilateral or bilateral Simultaneous or sequential ON Visual loss is severe Acuity severely reduced on follow-up May have uveitis also Outcomes are poor	CRION is usually • AqP-4 Antibody negative Rx: IV or oral steroids—initially good response, but • Later-on not such a good response • Long-term immunosuppression is needed
3.	Graves' disease	It is a potentially visual loss-causing condition • Proptosis + periorbital edema • Ocular myositis • Staring look Decreasing frequency of muscle involvement • LPS: Levator palpebrae superioris • IR • MR • SR • LR • Obliques	Seen in almost 50% patients with Graves' disease Most common extra-thyroid involvement of Graves' disease Also called • GED: Graves' eye disease • TED: Thyroid eye disease • Graves' ophthalmopathy
4.	NA-ION	Elderly >50 years Mild pain around eye (in 10%) Disc edema (segmental) Peri-papillary hemorrhages **Small cup-to-disc ratio**** s/o NA-ION	

9. CONGENITAL DISORDERS INVOLVING THE EYE

	Disorder	Clinical presentation	Cause, diagnosis and treatment
1.	CPEO Chronic progressive external ophthalmoplegia	Painless Progressive Symmetrical Ptosis + ophthalmoplegia But NO diplopia	Mitochondrial myopathy
2.	LHON Leber's Hereditary Optic Neuropathy	More in males Young males 20–40 years Sub-acute painless loss of vision • Sequential involvement of both eyes • Over weeks to months • **Central vision more affected** • **Colour** vision affected early • Optic atrophy is **late (>6 months)** Fundus: Circum-papillar telangiectasia NFL swelling around the disc FFA: Does not cause leakage from disc Rarely: Cerebellar ataxia • Myoclonus • Tremors • Movement ds • Muscle weakness • Distal sensory neuropathy • Migraine	Mitochondrial 3 mt mutations (90% cases) • 3460 • 11–77–8 • 1–44–84 Penetrance higher in men (50%) No effective Rx
3.	Harding's syndrome	Harding's syndrome = MS + LHON Unlike LHON—more common in females LHON occurs in a.w. MS—like illness • Severe visual loss • MRI s/o MS • Painless L/V	**T-14484-C**** mutation Mitochondrial genome

10. ION—ISCHEMIC OPTIC NEUROPATHY

a. ION = Sudden loss of vision due to interruption of blood supply to the optic nerve.

b. ION can be classified as

    i. Anterior ION: Involves the initial 1mm of ON (optic disc).

    ii. Posterior ION: Involves the optic nerve after the initial 1 mm (after disc). So, posterior ION will not cause disc edema.

c. Anterior ION has 2 types.

    i. Arteritic-Anterior ION: (A-AION): Caused by arteritis. Almost always GCA (giant cell arteritis).

    ii. Non-arteritic Anterior ION: (NA-AION) non-arteritis—Mostly idiopathic.

d. NA-AION

    i. NA-AION is the most common type of AION.

    ii. Usually presents in older patients >50 years.

    iii. Painless condition.

    iv. Although, pain may be seen in 10%.

    v. Anterior ION—so involves the disc: Causes disc edema, swollen hyperemic disc.

    vi. Peripapillary hemorrhages seen.

    vii. **Small disc-to-cup****ratio.

    viii. NA-AION has better prognosis than A-AION–70% improve.

	NA-AION (Non-Arteritis Ischemic Optic Neuritis)	A-AION (Arteritic-Ischemic Optic Neuritis)
Risk factors	Other than arteritis (vasculitis) • Idiopathic • Vascular • Drugs	Arteritis (vasculitis) • GCA: Giant cell arteritis • Temporal arteritis
Presentation	Acute Unilateral Painless Loss of vision Over hours to days	Acute Severe vision loss
Laterality	Unilateral	Unilateral/bilateral
Colour vision	May be normal	Abnormal
Vision loss	Less severe Usually, vision loss is less severe, so it is not possible to have No perception of light (PL)	More severe Patient may even have negative PL No PL—think of A-AION
Fundus angiography/ Fundus arteries	Normal Arteries are normal NA-AION may be due to venous insufficiency	Posterior choroidal Artery affected Posterior ciliary Artery occlusion
Disc	Normal or swollen disc Hyperemic	No blood supply, so Pallid disc
Visual field	Altitudinal defects	Dense central scotoma
Follow-up	Relatively preserved disc on resolution	Excavation or atrophy of disc
Disc hemorrhages	Common in NA-AION and CRVO (Both have a venous basis)	A-AION and CRAO—not common (Both have an arterial basis)
Diagnosis	Will have **all the signs and symptoms of optic neuropathy** • Reduced acuity • Dyschromatopsia • Field defects • Swollen Optic nerve • Splinter Hemorrhages • RAPD—relative afferent pupillary defect	

11. ABNORMAL VISUAL PHENOMENON

	Disorder	Clinical presentation	Cause, diagnosis and treatment
1.	CBS Charles Bonnet syndrome VRH Visual release hallucinations	Swiss philosopher Charles Bonnet described this phenomenon in his grandfather, who had vision loss due to cataract Patient has normal cognition but history of **Vision loss/Macular** degeneration (even 1 eye)	Rx: Treat the underlying cause Example: In cataract patients, hallucinations may improve after cataract surgery

(Continued)

(Continued)

	Disorder	Clinical presentation	Cause, diagnosis and treatment
1.	CBS Charles Bonnet syndrome VRH Visual release hallucinations (Cont'd)	• ARMD (age-related macular degeneration) • Cataract • Glaucoma C/P: Visual hallucination which are • Vivid, well-formed hallucinations • Realistic objects • More in evenings • MMSA/MoCA are normal • 10–15% in visual impairment • More in elderly	Medications • Quetiapine • Gabapentin • Escitalopram • Venlafaxine • Cholinesterase inhibitors
2.	Palinopsia	Disorder of visual perception in which there is • Persistence or recurrence of image • Even after the removal of stimulus • It gradually fades away in seconds–to–minutes As it is due to cortical lesions, palinopsia is associated with visual field defects	Due to **Post-geniculate cortical lesions**** from • Illicit drug use (LSD) • Migraine • Posterior circulation stroke • Vascular malformations • Tumours • Infections
		• Palinopsia with headache: Migraine • Palinopsia with normal examination: Illicit drugs • Palinopsia with visual field defects: See other causes of palinopsia	
3.	RVM Reversal of visual metamorphopsia	180-degree rotation of visual axis in CORONAL plane Everything is turned upside down It looks as if people are "walking on their heads" • Rare, transient phenomenon • Disappears soon	CT/MRI brain are normal Cause: Lesions of occipito-parietal regions • Brainstem or cerebellum • Migraine • Stroke • Head injury • Seizures
		Most common cause is Vertebro-basilar stroke Although, it can also be seen with tumours, vascular malformations, epilepsy	
4.	Peduncular hallucinations	Non-threatening hallucinations • Vivid • Colorful • Hallucinations of people, animals	Cause • Thalamus, Midbrain or pons lesions • Stroke • Osmotic demyelination • Inflammation • Infectious causes

	Disorder	Clinical presentation	Cause, diagnosis and treatment
5.	Pulfrich effect	2-D objects are perceived as 3-D It is basically a problem with depth perception The lateral motion of an object is perceived as having depth component • Trajectory of a tennis ball seems elliptical	Cause • Unilateral reduced vision (Optic Neuritis) • Decreased conduction velocity in 1 eye
6.	Poggendorf illusion	Geometrical-optical illusion • It involves the misperception of the position of one segment of a transverse line that has been interrupted by the contour of an intervening structure Just an optical illusion, no organic cause	 Figure 3.8 Interruption of the straight line by a grey tbox. The illusion is that the straight line is a continuation of red or the blue line.
7.	Abney effect	Hue shift or changes in hue of light Due to adding white light to monochromatic light source	
8.	Anton–Babinski syndrome	Visual impairment syndrome or visual anosognosia associated with denial of visual loss Impaired visual acuity But deny it (anosognosia) + confabulate **Cortical blindness****	 Figure 3.9 Lesion is a middle-aged woman with Anton–Babinski syndrome. Cause • Bilateral occipital lobe damage • Posterior cerebral artery infarction
9.	Balint–Holmes syndrome	Triad of • Optic ataxia • Oculomotor apraxia • Simultangnosia	Cause: Posterior parietal defects (bilateral)

(Continued)

(Continued)

	Disorder	Clinical presentation	Cause, diagnosis and treatment
10.	Apperceptive visual agnosia	Apperceptive visual loss • Impaired perception • Difficulty to identify objects • Difficulty in reproducing image • Copying image	Patient has normal • Visual acuity • Visual field • Colour vision Identify object with tactile or verbal perception
		• Matching image • Cannot identify clock • Cannot draw clock, overlapping pentagons	
11.	Associative visual agnosia	Associative agnosia Can copy objects But unable to identify the presented objects	
Characteristic and common ocular findings in neuro degenerative disorders			
12.	CBS Cortical basal syndrome	Slow saccades Slow saccadic pursuits Oculomotor apraxia Failure to initiate saccades Vertical EOM normal	
13.	PSP Progressive supranuclear palsy	Supranuclear gaze palsy Square wave jerks Apraxia of eyelid opening	
14.	MSA Multiple system atrophy	Blepharospasm excessive square wave jerks mild hypometria of saccades impaired VOR (vestibular-ocular reflex)	

DISORDERS OF PERIPHERAL NERVES, MOTOR NEURON AND MUSCLE

Part 1: Disorders of Peripheral Nerve and Motor Neuron

Abbreviations

- *AIDP*: Acute inflammatory demyelination polyradiculoneuropathy
- *ASO*: Anti-sense oligonucleotide
- *CIDP*: Chronic inflammatory demyelination polyradiculoneuropathy
- *C/P*: Clinical presentation
- *IVIG*: Intravenous immunoglobulin
- *MGUS*: Monoclonal gammopathy of unknown significance
- *NCS*: Nerve conduction studies

1. PERIPHERAL NEUROPATHY

Table 4.1   Differential Diagnosis of Neuropathy Based on Involvement

Pure sensory peripheral neuropathies	Pure motor neuropathies
<ul><li>Anti-MAG antibody neuropathy</li><li>CANOMAD</li><li>**Wartenberg migratory neuropathy**</li><li>**Cryoglobulinemia**—distal symmetrical sensory neuropathy</li></ul>	<ul><li>MMN/ MMN-CB (nerves involved: AIN, PIN, suprascapular nerve)</li><li>Lead poisoning</li></ul>
Predominantly sensory neuropathies	**Predominantly motor neuropathies**
<ul><li>Fabry disease</li><li>Amyloidosis</li><li>Sjogren's syndrome</li><li>Leprosy can have sensory neuropathies</li><li>Cryoglobulinemia—predominantly distal</li></ul>	<ul><li>Leprosy can have motor neuropathies</li></ul>
Symmetric motor weakness (proximal + distal)	**Symmetric proximal weakness**
<ul><li>AIDP, GBS</li><li>CIDP</li></ul>	<ul><li>Cervical or brachial diplegia</li><li>**Brachial amyotrophic diplegia**</li></ul>

(Continued)

DOI: 10.1201/b23306-4

Table 4.1   Differential Diagnosis of Neuropathy Based on Involvement (Continued)

Symmetric distal weakness	Asymmetric weakness
• CMT (HSMN)	• Mononeuritis multiplex
Upper limb onset/Predominant neuropathies	**Lower limb onset**
• Very few neuropathies start in upper limb • MMN/MMN-CB • Neuralgic amyotrophy • Hirayama monomelic amyotrophy • Cervical or brachial diplegia • Man in barrel syndrome • Lead neuropathy—wrist drop	• Most neuropathies are lower limb onset • Specially the axonal and length dependent

Anti-MAG Antibody Neuropathy

a. MAG = Myelin-associated glycoprotein.
b. Anti-MAG neuropathy is a slowly progressive neuropathy.
c. Predominantly sensory neuropathy (or sensori-motor).
d. Demyelinating neuropathy.
e. **Loss of vibration, joint position + ataxia.**
f. Most patient have MGUS > Waldenstrom Macroglobulinemia.
g. IgM monoclonal gammopathy (high serum IgM).
h. NCS: Prolonged velocities (demyelination type) in tested muscles.
i. **Rx: IVIG > Rituximab.**

CANOMAD

a. CANOMAD = Chronic Ataxic Neuropathy + Ophtahlmoplegia + IgM paraprotein + cold Agglutinins + Disialosyl antibodies.
b. C/P: Diplopia + Ophthalmoplegia + Distal paresthesia + Ataxia.
c. ~ Similar to MFS (Miller Fisher syndrome).
d. But CANOMAD very insidious and gradual progression (6 months).
e. Whereas MFS has an acute onset and progression.
f. Predominantly sensory neuropathy.
g. Motor nerves are grossly normal.
h. Investigations: Disialosyl Ab against GQ 1b, GT 1a, GD 1b.
i. Rx: IVIG and Rituximab.

> **BOX 4.1   FEATURES OF CANOMAD**
>
> • Distal to proximal gradient
> • Ataxia
> • Numbness
> • Fluctuating double vision
> • Joint position and vibration loss

Wartenberg Migratory Sensory Neuritis

a. Pure sensory neuropathy.
b. Recurrent mononeuropathy.
c. Sensory loss in one or more cutaneous nerves (recurrent episodes).
d. C/P: Pain/paresthesia/numbness in the distribution of sensory nerves.
e. Recurrent episodes.
f. Usually have a history of STRECHING of these nerves.
g. This disease may be associated with
    i. Diabetes mellitus.
    ii. HIV-AIDS.
    iii. Peripheral vascular disease.

CMT (Charcot–Marie–Tooth Disease)

a. **CMT = HSMN: Hereditary sensory motor neuropathy.**
b. Group of inherited neuropathies.
c. HSMN—neuropathy—so pattern of weakness is distal (lower legs and ankle first).
d. C/P: Childhood-onset disease.

Table 4.2   Clinical Features of CMT

Motor	Sensory	Others
Distal weakness: Difficulty in walking Bilateral pes cavus Atrophy of calf muscles	Glove and stocking sensory loss	Global areflexia Deformities Hammer toes High plantar arch

Classification of CMT

a. Based on the pattern of inheritance and type of neuropathy (axonal v/s demyelination)
   i. CMT 1: Autosomal dominant + Demyelination.
   ii. CMT 2: Autosomal dominant + Axonal neuropathy.
   iii. CMT 3: X-lined.
   iv. CMT 4: Autosomal recessive + Demyelination.
b. **Most common type of CMT = CMT1.**
c. **Most common type of CMT 1 = CMT 1a (70% of all CMT1, 50% of all CMT) = PMP22 mutation.**
e. CMT-3: Djerine–Sottas disease—Childhood onset, severe demyelination, mental retardation.

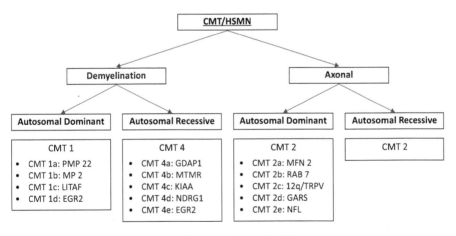

Figure 4.1   Genetic abnormalities in different types of CMT/ HSMN.

HNPP

a. HNPP = Hereditary neuropathy with pressure palsies.
b. HNPP is an inherited neuropathy.
c. Cause: PMP22 **Deletions** in 80%. PMP22 mutations cause CMT1a and PMP22 deletions cause HNPP.
d. Autosomal dominant disease.
e. Onset: In 20s–30s.

f. Recurrent acute sensory or motor disturbances in a single or multiple nerves.

g. Most common presentation: Peroneal neuropathy—foot drop.

h. Other pressure palsies include

    i. Ulnar nerve at elbow.

    ii. Median nerve at wrist.

    iii. Brachial plexus.

i. Prognosis: Patients show good recovery from pressure palsies.

j. Residual deficits are mild.

How to Say Whether There Is a Possibility of an Inherited Neuropathy or an Acquired Disease?

Table 4.3   Difference between Inherited and Acquired Neuropathies

Inherited neuropathy	Acquired neuropathy
Onset is earlier in life	Usually, onset is later in life
Family history positive	No family history
NCS: Uniform involvement	NCS: Patchy involvement may be seen • Patchy slowing • There may be conduction blocks and temporal dispersion in nerve conduction studies

MMN-CB

a. Multifocal motor neuropathy—with or without conduction block.

b. As the name suggests, it is

    i. Multifocal and asymmetric.

    ii. Motor predominant.

    iii. Starts in upper limbs.

> **BOX 4.2   MMN-CB**
>
> **Radial nerve palsy +
> Asymmetric atrophy (hand)**

c. Single nerve distribution (v/s dermatomal distribution in MND).

d. Fasciculations + (~similar to MND).

e. NCS: Conduction blocks ++.

f. CSF may show: High proteins but <1 g/dl.

g. 80% have GM1 antibody positive.

2. MOTOR SYSTEM DISORDERS

MND

a. MND = Motor neuron disease.

b. MND is not a peripheral neuropathy. It is an Anterior Horn Cell disease.

c. But is explained here, just to differentiate with MMN-CB.

Table 4.4   Difference between MND and MMN-CB

MND or ALS	MMN-CB
Anterior horn cell disease; dermatomal pattern	Peripheral neuropathy; nerve distribution
Asymmetric onset	Asymmetric onset
Upper motor neuron + lower motor neuron features	Only lower motor neuron features
Cramps + fasciculations ++	Cramps + fasciculations ++
Distal onset (hand weakness)	Distal onset (hand weakness)

MND or ALS	MMN-CB
Painless, no sensory symptoms	Painless, no sensory symptoms
Progressive	Progressive
Atrophy ++	Atrophy +
Tongue and bulbar involvement +	Rare
NCS—grossly normal	Conduction block +

Poor prognostic criteria for MND	Good prognostic factors
• Onset >80 years	• Onset <40 years
• Bulbar onset	• Spinal onset
• Definitive MND as per El Escorial criteria	• Long time between onset and diagnosis (slow progression)
• Poor FEV	

d. Drug of choice for Cramps: **Quinine.****

e. Other drugs for cramps: Quinine > baclofen > tizanidine/gabapentin/dantrolene.

f. Best predictor of respiratory function in MND: **Sniff Nasal Pressure.**

g. **5–10% MND patients may develop bvFTD** (behavioral variant of fronto-temporal dementia).

BOX 4.3   IMPORTANT POINTS ABOUT MND FOR EXAM

Q. Genetic or familial ALS: Most common—hexanucleotide repeats in non-coding region of C9orf

Q. 40% familial cases of MND are due to C9orf

Q. 10% develop FTD

SBMA (Kennedy Disease)

a. SBMA = Spinobulbar muscular atrophy.

b. Variant of MND.

c. Cause: Genetic—Trinucleotide repeat disease.

   i. Androgen receptor gene—trinucleotide expansion.

d. C/P

   i. Gynecomastia.

   ii. Oral and facial involvement.

   iii. Fasciculations ++.

   iv. Facial twitching.

   v. Reduced fertility.

   vi. **SENSORY nerve involvement.**

(D/b MND: MND is pure motor involvement; SMBA can have associated sensory involvement.)

SMA (Spinal Muscular Atrophy)

a. Genetic disease involving the central and peripheral nervous system.

b. Onset early in life.

c. There are 4 types of SMA described.

d. Most common SMA is SMA/SMN 1 (60%).

Table 4.5 Types of SMA

Types of SMA	Onset age	Clinical features	Prognosis
SMA-1: Congenital SMA	Before birth	Severe hypotonia; unable to sit; respiratory problems	Death within weeks
SMA-2: Werdnig–Hoffmann	<6 months	-Same-	Death in infancy
SMA-3: Dubowitz disease	6–18 months	Severe hypotonia; unable to sit/walk independently	Survives till adolescence
SMA-4: Kugelberg–Welander	Childhood/ Adolescence	May be able to walk	Survives till adulthood
SMA-5	Adult onset	Minimal motor deficits	Normal lifespan

e. A new genetic treatment is **Exondys 7.**
f. Omnasemnogene—gene replacement for **SMN 1—adenovirus 9**.
  i. Single IV dose.
  ii. Studies have shown that it improves ability to sit for 5 seconds in 92%.
g. Nusinersen = **Intrathecal.**
  i. Promotes the inclusion of **exon 7 during splicing of SMN** 2 gene.
  ii. Given intrathecal every 14 days × 3 doses.
  iii. Then 1 month later, then every 4 months.

3. AUTONOMIC SYSTEM NEUROPATHIES

AAG (Autoimmune Autonomic Ganglionopathy)

a. Acquired, immune-mediated disease.
b. Rare type of autonomic neuropathy.
c. Triggered by vaccines, viral illness and minor surgery.
d. Acute to sub-acute onset disease, pan-dysautonomia.
e. Progresses slowly over days to weeks.
f. Sympathetic + Parasympathetic involvement.
g. However, cholinergic involvement is more severe
  i. Dry eyes, dry mouth.
  ii. Dry bladder, dry gut.
  iii. Constipation, urinary retention.
h. **50% cases may have: ACHrR** Antibody positive.
i. **Others may have: Anti-Hu positive**—Paraneoplastic antibody.
j. **AAG having nACh-receptor positivity: Respond to IVIG.**

PAF (Pure Autonomic Failure)

a. More insidious onset.
b. Slower progression than AAG.
c. More likely to be degenerative rather than autoimmune.
d. PAF may herald alpha synucleinopathy by years. So patients should be followed by closely for development of parkinsonism.

POTS (Postural Orthostatic Tachycardia + Joint Hypermobility Syndrome)

a. Chronic orthostatic intolerance.
b. Increased HR (heart rate) within 10 minutes of upright posture.

   c. Patient feels: Palpitations, chest discomfort.

   d. Brain fog, blurred vision, intolerance, fatigue.

   e. Rx:

      i. Fludrocortisone.

      ii. Midodrine.

      iii. Pyridostigmine.

      iv. Propranolol.

Transthyretin Neuropathy

   a. Familial amyloid polyneuropathy.

   b. Autosomal dominant genetic disorder caused by transthyretin (TTR) gene mutations.

   c. Peripheral neuropathy + Autonomic neuropathy + Cardiovascular involvement.

   d. New approved drugs

      i. Patiseran.

      ii. Inoteseran.

      iii. ASO (anti-sense oligonucleotides) approved by FDA.

4. OTHER COMMON CLINICAL NEUROPATHIES

Mononeuritis Multiplex

   a. Rare, asymmetric peripheral neuropathy.

   b. Asymmetric involvement.

   c. Proximal and distal involvement.

   d. Multifocal involvement.

   e. Usually autoimmune in etiology.

   f. Causes: (see Box 4.4).

> **BOX 4.4   CAUSES OF MONONEURITIS MULTIPLEX**
>
> - Vasculitis
> - Lymphoma
> - Diabetes mellitus
> - Viral infections
> - Inflammation

Diabetes Neuropathies: Types

> **BOX 4.5   PATHOGENESIS OF DIABETES NEUROPATHIES**
>
> - Type 1 diabetes: Most important factor in pathogenesis is hyperglycemia. Hence, controlling hyperglycemia reduces neuropathy by 80%.
> - Type 2 diabetes: Rather than blood sugars, other metabolic disease parameters are also important in pathogenesis. For example: Abnormal lipids, obesity, hypertension.

   a. Most common type: Length dependent axonal neuropathy (50–70%).

   b. Mononeuropathies may be seen: Like carpal tunnel syndrome.

   c. Nerves are susceptible to compression.

   d. Diabetes amyotrophy.

   e. Autonomic neuropathy is less common.

   f. Radiculoplexopathy is uncommon.

   g. Treatment neuritis is uncommon.

   h. Diabetes-related proximal neuropathy is controversial.

   i. Diabetes-related CIDP has been reported in case reports and case series.

   j. Treatment of diabetes neuropathy—neuropathic drugs.

   k. Second-line–adjunctive = **alpha lipoic acid**—better than placebo.

BOX 4.6   DM AUTONOMIC NEUROPATHY

- Resting tachycardia +
- Diminished HR (heart rate) to oxidative stress
- Decreased CO (cardiac output)
- Orthostatic hypotension

**Orthostatic hypotension is related to mortality.

Cause: Vagus nerve denervation

BOX 4.7   DM AMYOTROPHY/ PLEXOPATHY

- Pain ++
- Weight loss ++
- Asymmetric + Proximal involvement
- Starts on one side (one leg), then spreads to other leg
- Proximal weakness ++ (predominant hip involvement)
- Muscle atrophy possible
- Sensory examination grossly normal
- Pathogenesis: Due to **micro-vasculitis****
- Ischemic nerve injury
- Prognosis: Slow recovery over 1–2 years

Inflammatory Radiculoneuropathies (AIDP/CIDP)

a. GBS = Guillain–Barré syndrome.
b. Clinical presentation
    i. Acute onset.
    ii. Asymmetric.
    iii. Proximal predominant weakness.
    iv. Ascending weakness (legs–trunk–upper limbs–bulbar and respiratory).
    v. May have sensory complaints at onset.
    vi. Back pain, burning parasthesia common.
    vii. Painful parasthesia.
    viii. However, bowel and bladder dysfunction is not seen.
c. Prognosis
    i. Probability of mobility @ 1, 3, 6 months based on 3 parameters (Box 4.9).
    ii. Age, antecedent infection and MMRC grade 3 weakness.
    iii. Modified ERASmus score can be used for same.
    iv. Increase in serum IgG **(delta IgG) at 2 weeks** can also be used.
    v. Patients with lower delta IgG have higher disability @ 6 months.
d. Investigations
    i. NCS: **SURAL sparing pattern**: classical of CIDP; may also be seen in AIDP.
    ii. CSF analysis: Albumin-cytological dissociation.
e. Treatment: IVIG and plasmapheresis
f. Sometimes, patient does not improve after the first dose of IVIG.
g. Whether second dose of IVIG has to be given to them—controversial topic.
h. Ongoing trial: SIDS GBS is evaluating the use of second dose of IVIG (Box 4.8).
i. There are many variants of GBS described in literature (see Table 4.6, Figure 4.2).
j. GQ1b antibody—positive in 80% of MFS cases.

BOX 4.8   SIDS-GBS

- SID = second dose of IVIG
In the SIDS GBS trial, second dose of IVIG (2 g/Kg) did not show any benefit in patients with poor prognosis (modified ERASmus score >6).

BOX 4.9   PROBABILITY OF MOBILITY IN GBS

- Age
- Antecedent diarrhea
- MMRC grade 3 weakness

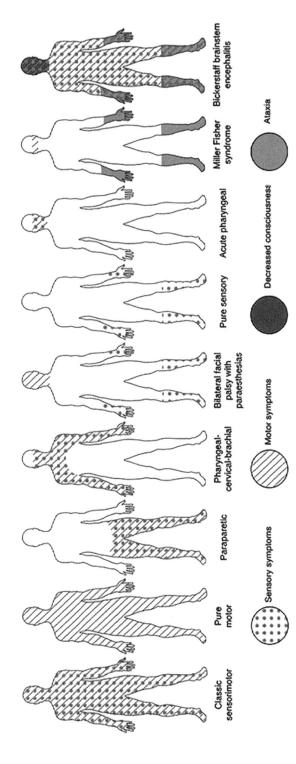

Figure 4.2 Variants of GBS/AIDP described in literature.

Table 4.6   Variants of GBS/AIDP

Neurophysiology variants	Regional variants
• AIDP • AMAN • AMSAN • Pure sensory variant	• Miller Fisher syndrome • Bickerstaff brainstem encephalitis • Cervical diplegia variant • Pharyngeal—cervical variant • Paraparetic variant

Concept of Nodo-Paranodopathies

a. The concept of nodo-paranodopathies has recently been described in cases of GBS.
b. There are demonstrable antibodies against specific antigens in nodes and paranodes of myelin sheath of a peripheral nerve.
c. This leads to dysfunction of nodes of Ranvier.
d. 10% GBS/CIDP patients: May have nodo-paranodopathies.
e. We should consider nodo-paranodopathies if
   i. **Distal predominant weakness (as opposed to proximal weakness in GBS/CIDP).**
   ii. **Prominent tremor (not seen in GBS/AIDP cases).**
   iii. **Sensory ataxia.**
   iv. **Poor response to treatment.**

BOX 4.10   EXAMPLE OF A CASE SCENARIO OF NODO-PARANODOPATHY WOULD BE

Q. 53-year-old woman presents with sub-acute progressive sensory-motor quadriparesis with distal-predominant sensory loss. A diagnosis of GBS/AIDP/inflammatory demyelinating polyradiculoneuropathy is considered. On examination, she also has hand tremors and sensory ataxia. NCS shows absent F waves, motor conduction block and a sural sparing pattern. She has not responded to IVIG, corticosteroids or plasmapheresis. How will you proceed?

i. In view of distal predominant weakness, ataxia, tremor—consider nodo-paranodopathies.
ii. Nodo-paranodopathies will respond to Rituximab.
iii. Also test for anti-MAG and monoclonal gammopathies.

Infectious Poly-Radiculitis

a. Presentation may be similar to mononeuritis multiplex.
b. Or polyradiculopathy (GBS/AIDP).
c. But CSF analysis will show increased cell count (pleocytosis).
d. Causes may include
   i. CMV (cytomegalovirus).
   ii. HIV–AIDS.
   iii. Lyme disease.

BOX 4.11   AN EXAMPLE OF A CASE SCENARIO OF INFECTIOUS
POLYRADICULITIS WILL BE

28-year-old woman has acute-onset progressive painless quadriparesis. NCS shows
asymmetric multifocal involvement. CSF shows increased protein and 50 cells.

Although the presentation may be thought of as AIDP or mononeuritis multiplex, the CSF
analysis shows 50 cells—pleocytosis.

The causes of CSF pleocytosis can be:
   i. Infectious polyradiculitis
  ii. Lymphoma
 iii. Meningeal carcinomatosis

Vasculitis and Vasculitis Neuropathy

Table 4.7   Common Vasculitis-Related Neuropathies

a. PAN Polyarteritis Nodosa	Medium vessel vasculitis Diagnosis requires 3/10 of ACR criteria Presence of Hepatitis B is one of the supporting criteria • Medium vessel vasculitis • Necrotizing vasculitis • Fibrinoid necrosis • Transmural inflammation • Weight loss • Asymmetric weakness, calf, EHL • Sensory loss, distal acrocynosis
b. ANCA vasculitis ANCA = Antineutrophilic Cytoplasmic Antibody	c-ANCA (proteinase 3): Granulomatosis with angiitis p-ANCA (MPO): Eosinophilic granulomatosis (Churg–Strauss syndrome) and microscopic polyangiitis If both c-ANCA and p-ANCA positive: May be a drug-induced vasculitis
c. Wegener's granulomatosis	Also called granulomatosis with angiitis Clinical features include: • Adult-onset asthma • Peripheral neuropathy • MPO (c-ANCA positive) • Eosinophilia in Peripheral smear • Multifocal neuropathy
d. Cryoglobulinemia	Symmetric distal sensory neuropathy Cryoglobulinemia triad • Generalized weakness • PALPABLE purpura • Diffuse joint pains Neuropathy features • Distal + symmetrical sensory • Small fiber predominant • Rarely multifocal

Toxic Peripheral Neuropathies

Table 4.8   Common Toxin-Related Neuropathies

a. **Sensory ganglionopathies**	Vitamin B6 excess (pyridoxine toxic neuropathy) Anti-cancer neuropathies • Cisplatin • Oxaliplatin • Carboplatin
b. **Motor neuropathies**	Lead causes motor predominant neuropathy Upper limb-onset neuropathy Wrist drop Foot drop
c. **Oxaliplatin**	Sensory ganglionopathy **Cold-induced hyperalgesia**** Cause: Increased neuronal excitability due to oxaliplatin effect on VGCC channels
d. **Ciguatoxin**	**Temperature inversion** **ciguatoxin is seen in** reef fish, barracuda, grouper, snapper Causes gastroenteritis + peripheral neuropathy Cold objects perceived as very hot
e. **Opioid-induced hyperalgesia**	**Diffuse allodynia**** Worsening pain with opioids Due to neuroplastic changes and opioid activation of inflammatory cells Sensitization of opioid receptors

Monoclonal Gammopathy

a. Monoclonal gammopathy of undetermined significance (MGUS) is a common benign precursor condition of multiple myeloma (MM) and related disorders.

b. MGUS is considered asymptomatic but has been shown to be associated with peripheral neuropathy.

c. Different types of neuropathies in MGUS/MM-related diseases

 i. CANOMAD.

 ii. POEMS.

 iii. Most common cause of neuropathy in MM = chemotherapy induced.

 iv. Serum VEGF levels are more than 5 times elevated in POEMS syndrome.

BOX 4.12   EXAMPLE OF A MONOCLONAL GAMMOPATHY-ASSOCIATED NEUROPATHY

A 55-year-old man has features of peripheral neuropathy and weakness of both feet. In next 5–6 months, he developed **foot drop** and **calf atrophy** with absent deep tendon reflexes. He also has skin **hyperpigmentation and hypertrichosis**, and hepato-splenomegaly with generalized lymphadenopathy. NCS shows a demyelinating neuropathy and serum VEGF levels are elevated.
• What is the diagnosis?
(Answer = POEMS syndrome.)

---

5. UPPER LIMB NEUROPATHIES

Neuralgic Amyotrophy

a. Idiopathic brachial plexo-neuropathy.

b. Uncommon and underdiagnosed condition.

   c. C/P
      i. New onset, sudden severe shoulder pain.
      ii. PEAKS in few hours.
      iii. Pain is not in the distribution of paresis.
      iv. Paralysis of muscles.
   d. The nerves commonly involved are: Long thoracic nerve.
   e. Supra-scapular nerve.
   f. AIN = Anterior interosseus nerve.
      i. Causes: Sensory loss in axillary nerve.
      ii. Paresthesia in the superficial radial and lateral antebrachial cutaneous nerve.
   g. Pathogenesis: Immune-mediated—Preceded by
      i. Infections.
      ii. Surgery.
      iii. Childbirth.
      iv. Mental strain.
   h. NCS may fail to show any abnormality.
   i. EMG: Shows denervation in the affected muscles.
   j. Rx: Oral prednisolone.
   k. Prognosis: Only 10% recover in 3 years.

Hirayama Monomelic Amyotrophy

   a. Also called oblique atrophy.
   b. Benign juvenile brachial spinal muscular atrophy.
   c. There is sparing of C5 and C6 muscles—so brachioradialis is spared.
   d. Involvement of C7, C8, T1 muscles.
   e. C/P: Insidious onset, Upper limb weakness.
   f. Usually asymmetric or unilateral onset.
   g. Onset in 20s and 30s.
   h. After years of progression—there is **a stationary phase**.
   i. NCS: Decreased CMAP in median and ulnar myotomes.
   j. EMG: Acute or chronic denervation in C7,C8,T1 myotomes.
   k. May require cervical cord MRI (in flexion and extension) for diagnosis.

Nerve root	Muscle groups	Muscles	Sensory	Reflexes
C5	Shoulder abduction Elbow flexion	Deltoid Biceps Brachialis	Lateral upper arm (deltoid patch)	Biceps reflex
C6	Elbow flexion Wrist extension	Biceps Brachialis Brachioradialis ECRL, ECRB	Outer aspect of forearm, thumb and index finger	Brachioradial/ Supinator
C7	Elbow extension Finger extension **Radial wrist flexion** **Wrist pronation**	Triceps Anconeus EPL, EPB EDC, EIP, EDQ FCR	Middle finger	Triceps
C8	Ulnar wrist flexion Finger flexion Hand grip	FCU FDS, FDP Thenar and hypothenar muscles	Ring finger and little finger Inner aspect of forearm	—
T1	Finger adduction Finger abduction	Interossei Lumbricals	Inner aspect of arm	—

Nerve	Muscle groups	Muscles	Sensory	Reflexes
Median	Wrist flexors Hand grip muscles Thenar muscles	FDS FDP (2nd and 3rd finger) FCR, palmaris longus Pronator quadratus	Palmar aspect of hand Lateral 3½ fingers	—
		Pronator teres Abductor pollicis brevis Flexor pollicis brevis Opponens pollicis Lumbricals 4th and 5th	Nails and tips of fingers on the dorsal aspect	
Ulnar	Ulnar deviation of hand Hand grip muscles Hypothenar muscles	FCU FDP (4th and 5th fingers) Adductor pollicis Flexor pollicis brevis Hypothenar muscles Lumbricals 3rd and 4th Interossei	Medial 1½ fingers	—
Radial	Elbow extensors Wrist extensors Finger extensors	Triceps Brachioradialis ECRL, ECRB	Majority of dorsal aspect of hand First dorsal web space	Brachioradial/ Supinator reflex

How to Differentiate Ulnar Neuropathy v/s C8 Neuropathy

a. Both C8 root and ulnar nerve supply muscles for ulnar wrist flexion and intrinsic muscles of the hand.
b. So, lesion in both will cause weakness of ulnar wrist flexion and
c. Weakness of intrinsic muscles.

However, the following clinical features may help in differentiating these entities.

C8 Root lesion	Ulnar nerve entrapment
Common features of both are: • Weakness of ulnar wrist flexion • Weakness of intrinsic muscles of hand	
Reduced sensation over medial forearm (medial antebrachial cutaneous nerve)	Sensory loss in the palmar aspect of 4th and 5th fingers
C8 root also gives some supply to the triceps muscle So, there may be some weakness of elbow extension and reduced triceps reflex	More prominent interossei and lumbricals weakness
C8-T1 roots also supply the median nerve innervated thenar muscles. There may be weakness of thenar muscles and weakness of flexion of inter-phalangeal joints of thumb	

C7 Root lesion	Radial nerve neuropathy
The common features of both are: • Weakness of elbow extension • Weakness of triceps muscle	
Reduced sensation over middle finger	Sensory loss in the dorsal web space Dorsal aspect of hand

C7 Root lesion	Radial nerve neuropathy
C7 prominently supplies triceps—so more pronounced triceps weakness and absent triceps reflex	Weakness of brachioradialis and wrist extension more prominent Absent brachioradial/Supinator reflex

Other Specific Entrapment or Compression Syndromes

Entrapment syndrome	Clinical features	Common differential diagnosis
Carpal tunnel syndrome— median nerve	Numbness and paresthesia over lateral 3 ½ fingers Thenar weakness No triceps weakness	**C6–7 radiculopathy** • C6–7 radiculopathy will have triceps weakness and will have sensory loss over the outer aspect of forearm
Cubital tunnel syndrome— ulnar nerve	Numbness and paresthesia over medial 1 ½ fingers Hypothenar weakness	**C8-T1 radiculopathy** (see previous table)
Posterior interosseus syndrome—radial nerve	Mainly motor weakness Wrist and finger extensor weakness Wrist and finger drop	**C7 radiculopathy** • C7 radiculopathy will have triceps weakness

6. PELVIC AND LOWER LIMB NEUROPATHIES

Diabetic Lumbosacral Amyotrophy

a. Mainly a Plexopathy (lumbar plexus involvement).
b. May be the 1st presentation of diabetes mellitus.
c. C/P: Painful condition.
d. Acute to sub-acute onset weakness of one leg (may involve the other leg later).
e. Severe PAIN. ++.
f. Proximal muscle weakness (thigh) with atrophy.
g. Associated with Significant weight loss >10 kg.
h. NCS: Profound reduction in CMAP (motor amplitudes).
   i. Reduced SNAP (sensory amplitudes).
   ii. Conduction velocities are only mildly affected.
   iii. EMG: Fibrillation potentials in paraspinal muscles.
i. Often co-exists with DSPN (distal symmetric peripheral neuropathy).
j. CSF: Raised protein levels—similar to root involvement.
   Raised CSF protein levels with normal cell count may also be seen in diabetes-related CIDP.
k. Rx: Painkillers, control diabetes.
l. Role of steroids is controversial. Steroids can cause further increase in blood sugar levels.
m. Can try IVIG.

Femoral Neuropathy

a. Injury or lesion of femoral nerve is an uncommon complication of surgical procedures.
   i. Lithotomy position during vaginal hysterectomy (less common).
   ii. Abdominal hysterectomy: Nerve caught b/w retractor and pelvic wall.
b. C/P: Leg weakness (thigh extension).
c. But thigh adduction normal.
d. Reduced sensation over medial and anterior thigh (intermediate cutaneous nerve and medial cutaneous nerves of thigh).

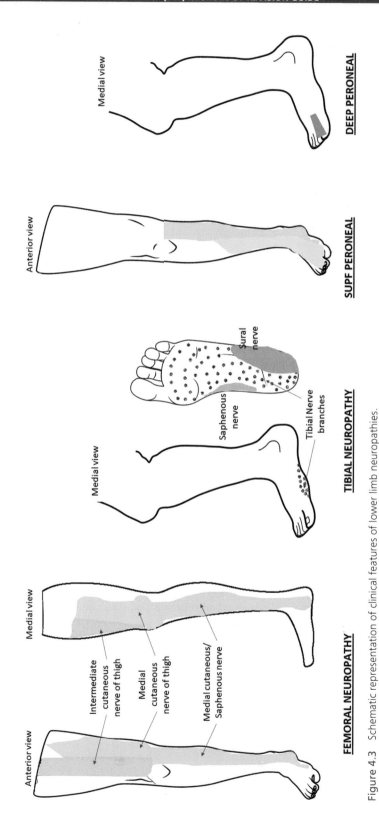

Figure 4.3   Schematic representation of clinical features of lower limb neuropathies.

Obturator Neuropathy

a. Obturator nerve is a large nerve travelling on the inner aspect of thigh.
b. It may be damaged during
    i. Forceps delivery.
    ii. Prolonged second stage of labour.
c. C/P: Weakness of the
    i. Adductor longus.
    ii. Adductor brevis.
    iii. Adductor magnus.
    iv. Gracilis.
    v. Pectineus.
    vi. Medial side/inner thigh sensory loss.

Specific Nerve Involvement in Lower Limb

Nerve	Motor weakness	Sensory loss
Femoral nerve neuropathy	Hip flexion weakness Knee extension weakness Absent knee reflex	Anterior and medial thigh Medial leg
Tibial nerve neuropathy	Ankle plantar flexion Ankle inversion Toe flexion	Medial and plantar aspect of sole
Superficial peroneal nerve	Foot eversion	Anterior leg and upper aspect of the foot
Deep peroneal nerve	Ankle dorsiflexion Toe dorsiflexion	Small part between the first and second toes

**Remember
- **LIED = L5—causes Inversion, Eversion, Dorsiflexion of foot (L-I-E-D)**
- **PED = Peroneal causes Eversion and Dorsiflexion**
- **TIP = Tibial causes Inversion and Plantar flexion**
- **Sciatic = Peroneal + Tibial**

How to differentiate between Sciatica + S1 Radiculopathy		
	Ability to tiptoe	Reduced ankle jerk
S1 Radiculopathy	No	Yes
Sciatica	No	No

How to differentiate between Peroneal neuropathy + L5 Radiculopathy				
	Foot drop	Able to invert foot	Ability to evert	Hip abduction weak
L5 Radiculopathy	Yes	No (tibial)	No	Yes
Peroneal neuropathy	Yes	Yes	No	No
Sciatica	Yes	No (tibial)	No	No

Localization of Foot Drop

Localization	Cause	Distinguishing point
CNS causes (brain)	Cerebral palsy	Congenital cause
	Stroke	Hemiparesis, aphasia
	Intracerebral hematoma	Spasticity
	Brain tumours Meningioma Metastasis	Headache, vomiting Raised ICP
Spinal causes	Spinal cord injury/Myelopathy	Spastic paraparesis
	L4–L5 root compression	Root pains Normal knee, Absent ankle reflex Difficulty in inverting/everting foot
Peripheral neuropathy Peroneal neuropathy	Trauma—fibula fractures, gunshots, iatrogenic-surgical	Definite history of the trauma P-E-D
	Compression due to splints Compression bandages Sitting crossed leg Prolonged kneeling	Loss of eversion and dorsiflexion Loss of sensation between 1st and 2nd toe space
	Internal compression due to compartment syndrome	
	Space-occupying lesions like Baker cyst, ganglion, lipoma, nerve sheath tumours	
Peripheral neuropathy Sciatic neuropathy	Compression at buttock Toilet seat Bed bound patients Intramuscular gluteal injections	Often peroneal involvement more severe than tibial involvement (PED > TIP) Loss of sensation on lateral calf and dorsum of foot
Others	Focal myopathies MMN-CB Lead poisoning	

DISORDERS OF PERIPHERAL NERVES, MOTOR NEURON AND MUSCLE

Part 2: Muscle Diseases

Abbreviations

- *ATS*: Andersen–Tawil syndrome
- *CMP*: Cardiomyopathy
- *EMG*: Electromyography
- *LGMD*: Limb Girdle muscle dystrophy
- *MD*: Muscular dystrophy
- *MUAP*: Motor unit action potentials
- *NCS*: Nerve conduction studies
- *PSW*: Positive sharp waves on EMG
- *SNHL*: Sensorineural hearing loss

1. IDENTIFYING FEATURES OF COMMONLY ASKED MUSCLE DISEASES IN EXAM

	Common identifying feature	Examples and D/D	Points in favor of specific myopathy and management of the condition
1.	Onset >40 years	a. OPMD (GCN repeats) Oculo-pharyngeal muscular dystrophy	Resident of Quebec, Canada, Bukhara Jews C/P: Ptosis, dysphagia Limitation of upgaze
			Genetics • Autosomal dominant, • Expansion of PABP-N1 • But NO anticipation • So patient has normal life span • Penetrance is age dependent
		b. IBM Inclusion body myositis	Usually, **ASYMMETRICAL** Or rarely may have Bilateral symmetrical weakness Mainly involves the **FF + KE** (finger flexors + knee extensors)

(Continued)

(Continued)

	Common identifying feature	Examples and D/D	Points in favor of specific myopathy and management of the condition
1.	Onset >40 years (Contd)		Quadriceps wasting is seen **In upper limb: FDS** involvement >> FDP No small muscle involvement
			EMG: Fibrillation, PSW seen, MUAP: Short-duration, small polyphasic potentials Antibodies: Anti-cytosolic-nucleotidase 1A Rx: Steroids are not used
		c. LGMD-1A	Limb girdle muscular dystrophy
		d. SLONM Sporadic late-onset nemaline myopathy	Biopsy shows: Sub-sarcolemma nemaline rods on Modified Gomori stain
		e. PMR Polymyalgia rheumatica	Most common rheumatological disease 10% PMR patients will have GCA (giant cell arteritis)
		f. Welander distal myopathy	Late-onset disease (>40 years) Distal myopathy Characteristic: Hand onset is classical of Welander Autosomal dominant Finger extension (long extensors) weakness Finger abduction weakness Small muscle wasting Genetics: TIA-1 mutation
2.	Prominent sexual features	Kennedy disease SBMA Spino-bulbar muscle atrophy	Onset in 20s–40s Mainly seen in Males Although it is a motor system disease, subclinical sensory symptoms may be + Sexual features (gynecomastia, inability to conceive) Fasciculations involving facial muscles Diabetes mellitus + CPK mild elevation only* Genetics: CTG repeats Normal life span* (same as OPMD)
3.	Presence of Diabetes mellitus (DM) in myopathy	a. Kennedy disease SBMA	(see previous)
		b. Myotonic dystrophy-1	Middle-aged man, Distal myopathy + ptosis + DM Myopathic facies: Hatchet face**
		c. MELAS mitochondrial disease	Onset in 20s–30s Multisystem disease Myopathy + DM + SNHL + short stature Symmetrical myopathy Biopsy and Gomori trichome staining shows: Ragged red fibres

	Common identifying feature	Examples and D/D	Points in favor of specific myopathy and management of the condition
4.	Distal-onset myopathy	a. Welander distal myopathy	Late-onset disease (>40 years) Distal myopathy—Hands involved Finger extension (long extensors) weakness Finger abduction weakness Small muscle wasting Genetics: TIA-1 mutation

2. DISTAL MYOPATHIES

The basic clinical difference between myopathies and neuropathies is that most myopathies and muscular diseases are proximal predominant diseases. That is why we have a limb girdle (shoulder girdle and hip girdle) involvement in muscle diseases. Conversely, most peripheral neuropathies are length-dependent. So, they involve the distal most parts like the hands and ankle and lower legs. However, that is not always true. There are certain primary muscle diseases, which can involve the distal muscles. To characterize the type of disease, we can use Figure 5.1.

3. MUSCLE DYSTROPHIES IDENTIFYING FEATURES

	Myopathy	C/P and important exam pointers	Clues to diagnose
1.	DMD Duchene muscular dystrophy and BMD: Becker MD	Starts in 1st decade of life DMD causes death by 20–25 years Pseudo-hypertrophy of calf The most common cause of death = **Cardiomyopathy**	Pediatric onset Pseudo-hypertrophy of calf Gower sign + Toe walking +
2.	LGMD 1c	Also called Caveolinopathy Autosomal dominant **Localized mounding** in muscles Rolling movements in muscle on tapping	Limb + Girdle weakness Proximal muscle weakness Percussion-induced ripples
3.	LGMD 2b	DYSFerlinopathy Inability to tiptoe Pseudo-hypertrophy of calf	
		DYSFerlinopathy has 2 clinical types a. LGMD 2b: Limb girdle type, autosomal recessive b. Miyoshi myopathy: Distal myopathy	
	Cardiac involvement is seen in LGMDs	• LGMD 1B • LGMD 2C, D, E, F • LGMD 2I	
	Mental retardation seen in	• LGMD 2M, N, O, P	
4.	Myotonic Dystrophy		
	Type 1	(CLUE: Muscle disease in a middle-aged man with involvement from eyes till hands with a typical hatchet facies) Ptosis + distal weakness + Everything in between • Facial and mastication weakness • Dysphagia, constipation Genetics: CTG repeats—DMPK gene	Middle-aged man Distal weakness Cardiac conduction Arrythmia Cognition abnormal Endocrinopathy Diabetes Facies
	Type 2	Proximal variant Genetics: Zinc finger protein 9	

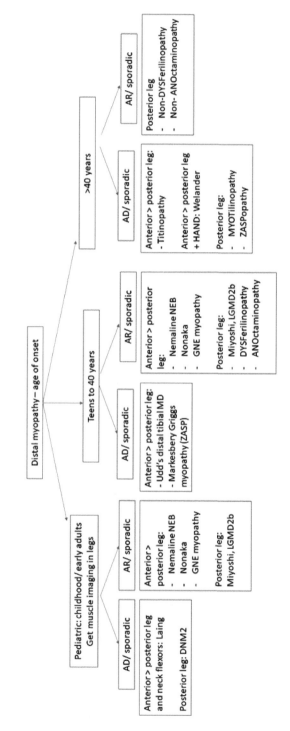

Figure 5.1

4. METABOLIC MYOPATHIES

a. All glycogen and Fatty acid oxidation (FAO) defects are Autosomal recessive except
- Phosphorylase b kinase deficiency.
- Phosphoglycerate kinase 1 deficiency.

b. Mitochondrial disease may be anything: Autosomal dominant, recessive, X-linked.

	Storage disease	C/P	Specific diagnosis
1.	GSD Glycogen storage disease	Exercise intolerance Second-wind phenomenon: 10 minutes of exercise produces improvement in exercise tolerance	GSD V—McArdle disease
		Out-of-wind phenomenon: Symptoms worsen with glucose/sucrose intake before exercise	PFK deficiency
		Hemolytic anemia along with GSD	GSD 7,9,12
		Mental retardation and dementia along with GSD	GSD 9,12 Adult polyglucosan disease
		Myogenic hyperuricemia	
2.	Lipid storage diseases	Fasting precipitates myalgia, weakness Prolonged exercise produces myalgia	

	Storage disease	C/F	Clues
1.	McArdle's	GSD V Autosomal recessive Myo-phosphorylase deficiency MC genetic myopathy Adolescent + exercise intolerance + second wind • Myalgia • Cramps, fatigue • Never good at sports • BUT RELIEF within few minutes • Sugar intake ameliorates symptoms Intense sustained exercise • Rhabdomyolysis • Myoglobinuria, AKI	Adolescent onset Second wind phenomenon CPK >1000 EMG: Fibrillation, myotonic Bx: Accumulation of glycogen—PAS staining Absent phosphorylase Vacuolated sarcoplasm
2.	Pompe's	Infantile form: Floppy baby + CMP Juvenile form: CMP is less common Adult form: Presents with respiratory weakness	
3.	Cori's	Distal muscle weakness + Polyneuropathy + Heart CMP hypoGLYCEMIA**	
4.	CPT II deficiency	Precipitated by • Prolong fast • Prolong exercise • Infections	CPT = Carnitine palmitoyltransferase
5.	VLCAD	Infancy onset—multisystem disease	VLCAD = Very long chain acyl-CoA dehydrogenase

5. MITOCHONDRIAL MYOPATHIES

	Storage disease	C/F	Clues
1.	KSS Kearns–Sayre syndrome	Onset <20 years with • EOM weakness • Pigmentary retinopathy + 1 of • Ataxia • Cardiac conduction abnormalities • CSF protein >100 mg/dL	
2.	MELAS	Onset <40 with • Atypical strokes • Migraine-like headache • DM, SNHL • Maternal inheritance	
3.	MERRF	• Maternal inheritance • Clinical triad of M-E-A • Myoclonus, epilepsy, ataxia	Myoclonus Epilepsy with Ragged red fibres
4.	CoQ10 deficiency	Proximal weakness High CPK, lactate	

6. MYOPATHIES WITH EARLY RESPIRATORY WEAKNESS

Mnemonic: "*I* Forgot *ADMINs r*elative"

I = **L**GMD 2i
F = **F**ukutin related
A = **A**dult-onset Pompe
D = **D**esminopathy
M = **M**yotonic dystrophy, mitochondrial ds
I = **I**nflammatory myopathy
N = **N**emaline myopathy

7. CONGENITAL MYOPATHIES

a. Present in Infancy—with floppy infant syndrome.
b. 10% of floppy infants have Congenital myopathy.
c. Other clinical features: Hypotonia + Muscle weakness.
d. Usually have a Slow progressive or static course.
e. Diagnosis is based on biopsy.
  i. Ryanodine central cores or core rods.
  ii. Nemaline NEB rods.
  iii. Dynamin centro-nuclear or myotubular.
  iv. Fibre disproportion with type 1 hypotrophy.

	Myopathy	C/F	Clues
1.	RyR central core	RyR-1 • Decreased fetal movements • Breech presentation • Floppy infant • Delayed milestones • CDH + pes cavus + planus + clubfoot + scoliosis • Arthrogryposis • Kyphoscoliosis	Initial ocular + Facial + Skeletal abnormality Family h/o MHS **Biopsy: Type 1 predominant Central cores**
		Malignant hyperthermia syndrome (MHS) is allelic disease to RyR core disease	

	Myopathy	C/F	Clues
2.	RyR diseases spectrum (allelic diseases)	a. RyR Central core disease (AD) b. MHS: Malignant hyperthermia c. Rhabdomyolysis	
		RyR-related rhabdomyolysis • Muscle hypertrophy • Superior athletic ability • Run long walks, marathons • But may develop rhabdomyolysis, AKI (acute kidney injury) • Family h/o sudden death/weakness	Family h/o Myalgias Heat intolerance
3.	Nemaline rod disease	NEB in 50% ACTA-1 in 25% Facies similar to congenital MD • Long narrow face • Prognathous • Early respiratory involvement	
4.	SLONM Sporadic, late-onset nemaline myopathy	Congenital myopathy, but clinical presentation is late in life Progressive weakness + severe atrophy of all muscles • Upper Limb, Lower Limb • Axial muscles + • Neck drop + • Respiratory weakness 50% have IgG-MGUS Rx: 1/3 patients respond to steroids Others may need stem cell transplant	Late onset Head drop All muscles, atrophy **IgG-MGUS** **NORMAL CPK****** **Bx: Nemaline rods**
5.	HIV-NM	HIV-associated nemaline myopathy Same as other nemaline myopathies, BUT • No facial weakness • No respiratory weakness	**Biopsy: Type 1 predominance Selective atrophy of type 1 Deficiency of 2B Sub-sarcolemmal red staining rods**
6.	Centronuclear	Dynamin DNM2 gene Ptosis + face weakness	
7.	Myotubular congenital myopathy	MTM-1: X-linked gene Variant of centro-nuclear myopathy • Infancy onset • Decreased fetal movements • Polyhydroamnios • Floppy infant • Hypotonia • Respiratory weakness	X-linked Undescended testis Inguinal hernia Pyloric stenosis **Bx: Triad of** • **Type 1 predominant** **Type 1 hypertrophy** • **Increased central nuclei** • **Radiating sarcoplasmic strand**

(Continued)

(Continued)

	Myopathy	C/F	Clues
8.	Fibre type disproportion	ACTA-1 gene Type 1 hypotrophy • High arch palate • Ankle contracture • CDH	
9.	Multi-minicore disease	SEPN (selenoprotein) • Axial involvement • Spine rigidity • Scoliosis • Respiratory weakness	
10.	Core-rod disease	RyR-1 gene	

8. PERIODIC PARALYSIS (PP) AND CHANNELOPATHIES

a. Autosomal dominant diseases.
b. 1st and 2nd decade onset.
c. Except TPP; which is 3rd and 4th decade.
d. Episodic weakness after triggers.
e. Channelopathy
   i. Hypokalemic PP = Calcium.
   ii. Hyperkalemic PP = Na/sodium.
   iii. ATS = K/potassium channels.
f. Types of attacks
   i. Maximum number of attacks in hyperKalemic PP = short attacks (last < 1 hour).
   ii. Longest attacks in TPP = last for days.
   iii. Most severe attacks = hypoKalemic PP – later in life leads to weakness.
   iv. Myotonia only in hyperKalemic PP (out of the main 4 types of PP).
g. Rx for all 3 is potassium (K+) supplementation, except hyperKalemic PP.
h. Insulin + dextrose for hyperKalemic PP, IV calcium gluconate is also used.
i. **Beta-blockers for** thyrotoxicosis (Drug of Choice).**
j. Inhaled beta-blockers can be used for hyperKalemic PP.

	Periodic Paralysis (PP)	Clinical features	Clues
1.	HyperKalemic PP Na channel SCN4a gene	Children <20 years present with • Paralytic episodic attacks after • Exercise • Cold exposure • Potassium-rich food • Emotional stress • Pregnancy • Attacks are short: Last few minutes to 1 hour • Stiffness maybe present between attacks Rx: Heavy meal (Carbohydrate-rich) before exercise **Acetazolamide**, Dichlorphenamide reduces frequency **Salbutamol** 1–2 puff shortens the attack	• <20 years • Cold-induced • Exercise-induced • (~PMC) • ECG: Tall T waves

	Periodic Paralysis (PP)	Clinical features	Clues
2.	HypoKalemic Ca channel CACNA1s SCN4a KCNE	Same as hyperKalemic PP <20 years onset Muscle paralysis after: • A heavy Carbohydrate-meal Flaccid paralysis: • On awakening @night or early morning Long-lasting attack: Lasts for hours** Spares respiratory and bulbar muscles **Autosomal dominant, reduced penetrance** in women So may not get family h/o (if mother has hypokalemic PP) Most important D/D is GBS: • There is sparing of respiratory and bulbar muscles in hypokalemic PP	<20 years CHO meal-induced Exercise-induced Longer attacks Blood tests: Serum K+ levels low ECG: Absent T waves, presence of U waves
3.	ATS Andersen–Tawil syndrome K channels KCNJ2 Kir 2.1	Triad Episodic weakness Facial dysmorphic — Ventricular arrythmia Figure 5.2 Short stature, low-set ears, hypertelorism, micrognathia, clinodactyly, syndactyly	ECG: Prolonged QTc Blood tests: Serum K may be low, normal or high
4.	TPP Kir 2.6 KCNj8	Thyrotoxic periodic paralysis	Thyrotoxicosis
5.	MC Myotonia congenita	Myotonia but no muscle weakness Herculean appearance* Patient has a Muscular build Myotonia improves with exercise: "WARM UP" Men more severely affected There are 2 types of MC { Thomsen MC / Becker MC table below }	Chromosome 7 CL.CN1 mutations

Thomsen MC	Becker MC
AD autosomal dominant	AR recessive
Infancy onset	Late childhood onset
Face and UL onset	Lower limb onset
Less severe disease	More severe
No atrophy	Some atrophy seen later
SET: No decrement	Initial decrement +
Fournier pattern III	II

(Continued)

(Continued)

	Periodic Paralysis (PP)	Clinical features	Clues
6.	PMC Paramyotonia congenita Von-Eulenberg disease SCN4a	Autosomal dominant Episodic cold-induced myotonia Episodic exercise-induced myotonia Paradoxical myotonia—increases with repeated muscle activity May resemble hyperKalemic PP in episodic attacks of paralysis Classical C/P • Frozen smile, frozen tongue • Involuntary eye closure after washing face • Frozen smile in winters • Frozen tongue after ice cream • Child is not really muscular (d/b MC) • SET/LET: significant decrement Rx: CBZ, PHT (antiepileptic drugs) • Mexiletine, Flecainide	Cold-induced Exercise-induced Eyelid myotonia Washing face cold water Ice cream, winters
		*PMC is allelic with SCN4a diseases *Muscle stiffness in PMC worsens with exercise (rather than improve)	
7.	KAM/PAM Potassium aggravated myotonia Na channel	Myotonia not aggravated by cold No prominent weakness 3 types • Myotonia fluctuans • Acetazolamide responsive • Myotonia permans	
8.	SJS Schwartz–Jampel syndrome	Chondro-dystrophic myotonia • Myotonia + • Bone dysplasia + short stature + • Dwarf + contractures • Microstomia, poor facial expression • Skeletal: Pes, coxa, dysplasia	Crouched gait Waddling gait Dwarf child

9. NON-DYSTROPHIC MYOTONIA

a. Myotonia+ but no major muscle weakness (no dystrophy, no muscle weakness).
b. Examples: MC, PMC, hyperKalemic PP, SJS, KAM.
c. MC (Myotonia Congenita) has 2 types: Thomsens or Beckers.
d. Rx for myotonia
   • Anti-myotonia agents.
   • Mexiletine.
   • Clomipramine, imipramine.
   • CBZ, procainamide, Acetazolamide.
   • Lacosamide and ranolazine are upcoming drugs.

10. FOURNIER PATTERNS: (SET/LET)

I: Significant decrement >60s: PMC (Paramyotonia congenita).
II: Decrement <60s, then recovers: Becker MC.
III: No decrement: Thomsen MC.
IV: Increment.

(SET: Short Exercise Test/LET: Long Exercise Test)

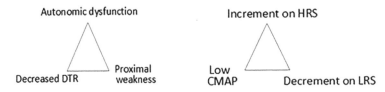

Figure 5.3   Clinical and electrophysiological triads of LEMS.

11. LAMBERT–EATON MYASTHENIA SYNDROME (LEMS)

a. Pathogenesis: P/Q type voltage gated calcium (VGCC)—Cav 2.1
b. Clinical triad (P-A-D).
c. Electrophysiological triad.
d. *Starts in LL (lower limbs).*
e. Main presentation maybe fatigue.
f. DTR are absent in 90–100%.
g. But for a short time: increased DTR may be seen after exercise.
h. This is called "**Post-exercise facilitation**".
i. Also transient increase in fatigue and muscle strength.
j. Autonomic features: Dry mouth, Erectile Dysfunction, constipation.
k. Altered sweating, postural hypotension, blurred vision.
l. Most common autonomic feature: **Dry mouth.****
m. There are 2 types of LEMSs.

T-LEMS (Tumour-associated LEMS)	NT-LEMS (Non-tumour-associated LEMS)
Age of onset 60 years	Onset in young: 30–35 years
Seen in Smokers	Non-smokers
Males > females	M = F
Associated with lung cancer: SCLC	—
Distal weakness may be seen	—
Respiratory weakness may be seen	—
Sensory dysfunction may develop	—
Ataxia may develop	—
High DELTA-P score	Low score

DELTA-P score	Points
Bulbar involvement (dysarthria, dysphagia)	1
Erectile dysfunction in men	1
Loss of weight >5%	1
History of tobacco use (at onset)	1
Age at onset of symptoms >50 years	1
Karnofsky performance status <70	1
• Score of 0 or 1: 0–2.6% chance of SCLC (almost excluded SCLC as a cause) • Score of 4, 5, 6: 93%, 96%, 100% chances of SCLC	

Diagnosis

a. Voltage-gated Calcium channel: VGCC IgG-Antibody + in 90%.
b. High-frequency RNS (50 Hz): Incremental response.
c. Short exercise test: CMAP improve by 100%.

Rx

a. Main aims is to reduce quantal release of Ach.
b. 3,4-DAP (Diaminopyridine) is used.
c. Blocks pre-synaptic VGCC.
d. Increases Acetylcholine release.
e. Steroids and AZA (azathioprine) may be used.
f. Screen for tumours in all suspected cases of LEMS especially lung cancers.

12. MYASTHENIA GRAVIS-LEMS OVERLAP

a. Prominent oculo-bulbar symptoms, AChR antibody positive.
  - But decreased DTR + electrophysiological triad of LEMS + VGCC +

DISORDERS OF THE SPINAL CORD

Abbreviations

- *ASIA scale*: American SCI Association Impairment scale
- *C/P*: Clinical presentation
- *LETM*: Longitudinally extensive transverse myelitis
- *MND*: Motor neuron disease
- *NMO-SD*: Neuromyelitis optica spectrum disorders
- *SACD*: Sub-acute combined degeneration of spinal cord
- *SCI*: Spinal cord injury
- *SMA*: Spinal muscular atrophy
- *VHL*: Von Hippel–Lindau syndrome

1. SPINAL CORD SYNDROMES

1. Pure dorsal column syndrome	2. SACD: Dorsal + lateral column syndrome	3. Central cord syndromes
Tabes dorsalis (syphilis) Treponema pallidum Tertiary syphillis Hemangioblastoma (VHL)	Vitamin B12 deficiency Vitamin E deficiency Copper deficiency HIV vacuolar myelopathy HTLV-1 virus myelopathy Adrenomyeloneuropathy	Typically seen in Syringomyelia Upper limb weakness >>> Lower limb Suspended sensory level Shawl-like sensory loss
4. Anterior horn cell syndrome	**5. Anterior spinal cord syndrome**	**6. LETM**
MND SMA Poliovirus Flavivirus: West Nile virus	Infarction of ASA • Thoracic abdominal **aorta aneurysm** repair • **Fibro-cartilage embolism**	NMO-SD Beçhet's disease Sarcoidosis Sjögren's syndrome B12 deficiency

2. CERVICAL SPINAL CORD INJURY

High cervical SCI	Low cervical SCI
Trunk anhidrosis seen Interrupt descending pathways to inter-medio lateral horn	Quad breathing Preserved diaphragm, but paralyzed thoracic and abdominals
Sympathetic fibres are damaged—so there is neurogenic shock Unopposed parasympathetic vagal activity Bradycardia, hypotension	Chest moves in, abdomen moves out

DOI: 10.1201/b23306-6

Poor Prognostic Factors in Cervical Myelopathy

a. Older age.

b. Gait impairment.

c. High myelopathy score.

d. T1 low and T2 high signal in MRI cervical spine.

3. SPECIFIC SPINAL CORD DISEASES

	Disease	Clinical presentation and pathogenesis	Diagnosis and treatment
1.	ASA infarction: Anterior spinal artery infarction	Rare and devastating disease C/P • Back pain in 70% • Motor weakness + areflexia • **loss of pain and temperature** • **Preserved joint position and vibration** (dorsal column) • Bladder and bowel involvement + • Initial signs are due to spinal shock Later on may develop spastic paraparesis	MRI spine Diffusion restriction in the area of infarction Treat with anti-thrombotics Treat the underlying cause Prognosis is guarded.
		Most common cause: Thoracic abdominal **aorta aneurysm** repair (4–30%) Mechanism: Embolism/segmental occlusion of arteries, distal aortic perfusion pressure Other causes • Vascular (cardioembolic) • **Fibro-cartilage embolism** (young + exercise) ASA embolism is rare in proximal diseases (cardiac, aortic). These diseases cause more of cerebral embolism	
2.	Copper deficiency myelopathy	Presentation similar to SACD (see later) Cause • Bariatric surgery • Zinc supplements	Diagnosis by MRI spine
3.	Vitamin B12 deficiency	SACD Sub-acute combined degeneration of spinal cord Combined = Lateral + posterior columns • Lateral column: Cortico-spinal tract: Spastic-ataxic paraparesis • Posterior column: Dorsal columns: loss of joint position and vibration • Myeloneuropathy • UMN + LMN signs	Diagnosis: MRI spine Blood tests: Low B12 levels B12 deficiency symptoms may be present even with borderline normal B12 levels. In that case, we should do Homocysteine and Methymalonyl acid levels They will be high because vitamin B12 is required for conversion of these In cystic fibrosis: **Fat-soluble vitamins—Vitamin E deficiency**

	Disease	Clinical presentation and pathogenesis	Diagnosis and treatment
		There may be other manifestations of B12 deficiency: • Anemia • Hyper pigmentation of knuckles • Cognitive deficits—memory loss • Fatigue and depression • Gastrointestinal issues	
4.	Beçhet's disease	Chronic + relapsing disease C/P • Oral + genital + ocular + skin lesions • 50% have CNS involvement— • **Basal ganglia + brainstem involvement** • 10% have spinal cord—**LETM** The classical clinical triad is Oral + Ocular + genital ulcers	MRI brain: Basal ganglia + brainstem involvement Pathergy test can be used for diagnosis Rx: Immune suppression
5.	Spinal DVAF Dural Arterio-venous fistula	Most common encountered vascular malformation of spinal cord and easily treatable DAVFs cause symptoms through venous hypertension and congestion of the cord with edema. Most common clinical presentations is progressive pain, lower extremity weakness or sensory changes Sphincter dysfunction may also occur	MRI spine: Look for presence of flow voids Steroids worsen symptoms in 50% Surgery better than embolization Lesser recanalization rates in surgery Otherwise, recovery same in both (surgery/embolization)
6.	Toxin/Toxic myelopathies	a. NO • NO = Nitric Oxide • NO causes SACD like presentation • Involvement of lateral column + dorsal column • NO related myelopathy is seen in whipped crème canisters • NO also causes irreversible inactivation of B12 • So urgent B12 supplementation is required for treatment b. Heroin • Heroin causes acute flaccid para/quadriparesis • This may be an immune-mediated phenomenon c. Manganese toxicity—causes parkinsonism-like presentation d. Check point inhibitors (anti-cancer drugs): Cause myelopathy—present as Transverse myelitis	

(Continued)

(Continued)

	Disease	Clinical presentation and pathogenesis	Diagnosis and treatment
7.	Infectious myelopathies	EBV (Epstein–Barr Virus): Spinal Cord syndrome + lymph-adenopathy + sore throat + headache + fatigue Flavivirus: West Nile virus-related myelopathy—Areflexia with weakness (presentation is similar of Anterior horn cell disease). MRI shows ventral cord enhancement + root enhancement Schistosoma-related myelopathy: treatment is with steroids and praziquantel Treponema infections: Tertiary syphilis—presents with posterior column involvement. MRI spine shows T2 hyperintense and nonenhancing lesions in posterior column In HIV-AIDS with CMV infection: CMV may cause lumbosacral polyradiculopathy, which resembles cauda equina syndrome	
8.	SCI while **intoxication**	Any patient who has a traumatic spinal cord injury while in an intoxicated state: NICE guidelines recommend that **Neck** immobilization should always be done, irrespective of neurological deficits, as neurological examination is unreliable	
9.	HSP **Hereditary spastic paraparesis**	**HSPs are a large group of inherited myelopathies** The prominent clinical symptom is difficulty in walking Clinical examination is remarkable for gross lower limb spasticity but mild weakness A large number of genes have been discovered for different types of HSP Complicated HSP = When HSP presents with additional neurological symptoms like: • Ocular symptoms • Optic dysfunction • Cognitive deficits • Peripheral neuropathy	MRI spine may be normal or show cord atrophy Genetic analysis may be done: a. Spastin: SPG-4 mutations: Responsible for 40% of cases • SPG-4 is the most common cause of Autosomal Dominant adult-onset HSP MRI brain: In SPG-11 and SPG-15 mutation—MRI brain may show a classical **"Ear of Lynx" sign** with thin Corpus Callosum
10.	LOFA **Late-onset Friedreich Ataxia**	(See next chapter for more details) Normal age of onset of Friedreich Ataxia: <25 years LOFA: Late onset ≥25 years VLOFA: Very late onset ≥40 years The age of onset may depend on the number of trinucleotide repeats • Lower number of trinucleotide repeats: GAA • Lesser number of repeats—less severe disease—late onset Patients have more spasticity, more hyperreflexia But less cardiomyopathy Usually there is minimum or no ataxia—so difficult to diagnose. So, diagnoses mainly depend on clinical suspicion, family history and genetic testing	

	Disease	Clinical presentation and pathogenesis	Diagnosis and treatment
11.	Post-radiation syndromes	**Post-radiation myelopathy**	**Post-radiation LMN syndrome**
		Onset may be acute in days to weeks or after 6 months More white matter demyelination >> rather than edema Spinal atrophy Usually irreversible	Delayed onset • 10–20 years later Distal Spinal cord and cauda equina involvement Secondary to • Testicular Cancer • Lymphoma • Vertebral metastasis
		• UMN syndrome	• Pure motor syndrome—LMN features • Fasciculations, absent reflexes • MRI: Lumbo-sacral nodular enhancement

4. CAUDA AND CONUS SYNDROMES

  a. Both cauda equina and conus medullaris syndromes are neurological emergencies.
  b. They can present with
  - Back pain radiating to the legs.
  - Motor and sensory dysfunction.
  - Bladder and/or bowel dysfunction.
  - Sexual dysfunction and saddle anesthesia.

	Conus medullaris syndrome	Cauda equina syndrome
Anatomy	Lower, conical part of the spinal cord	Nerve roots exiting from the spinal cord
Type of syndrome	UMN + LMN	LMN
Level of lesion	L1–L2/3	L2–sacral
Onset	Sudden Bilateral, symmetrical	Gradual Unilateral or asymmetric
Low back pain	More pain	Less pain
Radicular pains	Not seen	++
Motor	Paraparesis Symmetrical UMN type, spastic	Asymmetric or unilateral weakness LMN type Flaccid
Reflexes	Hyper reflexia	Diminished reflexes
Sensory loss	Symmetrical Peri-anal numbness	Asymmetrical Saddle anesthesia
Impotence	++	Uncommon
Bowel and bladder	Early dysfunction Bowel and bladder incontinence	Late and less common Urinary retention
Most common cause	Prolapsed inter-vertebral disk	

   c. Generally, we diagnose spinal cord syndromes by clinical examination and MRI spine. However, a nerve conduction study may be done. The electrophysiological differences in myelopathy (UMN weakness) v/s cauda equina (LMN weakness) are

      i. Both can cause sensori-motor paraparesis.

      ii. Sensory NCS (nerve conductions) are normal in both (both are pre-ganglionic involvement).

      iii. EMG: Cauda equina syndrome may have neurogenic motor units (polyphasic, increased amplitude and duration). Myelopathy patients will have normal EMG.

5. ASIA SCALE LEVELS

   a. *Sensory level*: Most caudal level—intact for BOTH pain and light touch.

   b. *Motor level*: Lowest level that has muscles with power—MMRC grade 3/5, till the upper level has 5/5.

   c. *Neurological level*: Most cephalad of the motor or the sensory level.

NEURO-GENETICS

Abbreviations

- *AD*: Autosomal dominant
- *ALS/MND*: Amyotrophic lateral sclerosis/Motor neuron disease
- *AR*: Autosomal recessive
- *CMP*: Cardiomyopathy
- *DM*: Diabetes mellitus
- *DTR*: Deep tendon reflexes
- *ECG*: Electrocardiography
- *NCS*: Nerve conduction studies
- *SCA*: Spinocerebellar ataxia
- *SNAP*: Sensory nerve action potentials
- *LL*: Lower limb
- *UL*: Upper limb
- *VOR*: Vestibulo-ocular reflex

1. INHERITED AND CONGENITAL DISEASES

* Most common cause of inherited intellectual disability: FXTAS

	Disease	Clinical presentation	Diagnosis and treatment
1.	FA Friedreich ataxia (Diagnostic criteria given by Anita Harding)	Diagnostic criteria (Harding) Essential for diagnosis • Onset <25 years • Progressive ataxia • Absent DTR in LL • Extensor plantar (Babinski sign) • Axonal sensory neuropathy • Dysarthria (after 5 years) Secondary/Additional features (seen in 66%) • Pyramidal weakness in LL • Absent DTR in upper limbs • Scoliosis • ECG changes • Distal loss of position and vibration Less common • Nystagmus • Optic atrophy	Trinucleotide repeat disorder Genetic analysis: Chromosome 9 • Frataxin gene • AR disorder • GAA repeats 20% (10–30%): have DM 60%—have CMP 70%—have scoliosis 70%—have pes cavus 90%—have dysarthria

(Continued)

DOI: 10.1201/b23306-7

(Continued)

	Disease	Clinical presentation	Diagnosis and treatment
1.	FA Friedreich ataxia (Diagnostic criteria given by Anita Harding) (Contd)	Normal age of onset of Friedreich Ataxia: <25 years LOFA: Late onset ≥25 years VLOFA: Very late onset ≥40 years The age of onset may depend on the number of trinucleotide repeats • Lower number of trinucleotide repeats: GAA • Lesser number of repeats—less severe disease—late onset Patients have more spasticity, more hyperreflexia But less cardiomyopathy Usually there is minimum or no ataxia—so difficult to diagnose. So, diagnoses mainly depend on clinical suspicion, family history and genetic testing	
2.	CANVAS: Cerebellar Ataxia Neuropathy Vestibular Areflexia Syndrome	Cerebellar ataxia + neuropathy + vestibular areflexia CANVAS disease has all 3 pathogenic mechanisms of ataxia 3 foci of ataxia • Cerebellar: Limb and gait ataxia • Sensory ataxia: (mainly ganglionopathy)* • Vestibular ataxia Onset is Late C/P: >50 years (~FXTAS) Characteristic sign is: **Impaired VISUALLY ENHANCED VOR** • Combined impairment of • VOR • Smooth pursuit • Optokinetic reflex Auditory functions are preserved** Autonomic symptoms • Cold feet • ED—erectile dysfunction • Constipation • Light headedness	**MRI brain: Atrophy of vermis** Mainly anterior and dorsal cerebellar vermis NCS: Absent SNAPs
3.	HSP Hereditary spastic paraplegia	Familial spastic paraplegia Group of inherited disorders causing UMN/spastic weakness mainly of the lower limbs Spasticity >>> weakness The prominent clinical symptom is difficulty in walking Clinical examination is remarkable for gross lower limb spasticity but mild weakness A large number of genes have been discovered for different types of HSP.	MRI spine may be normal or show cord atrophy Genetic analysis: a. Spastin: SPG-4 mutations: Responsible for 40% cases • SPG-4 is the most common cause of Autosomal dominant adult-onset HSP SPG-11 and SPG-15 disorders Autosomal recessive HSP MRI: Ears of the lynx sign Thinning of corpus callosum on sagittal sections

	Disease	Clinical presentation	Diagnosis and treatment
		Complicated HSP = When HSP presents with additional neurological symptoms like: • Ocular symptoms • Optic dysfunction • Cognitive deficits • Peripheral neuropathy Mainly spinal cord abnormalities are expected; however, MRI brain may also show some changes	

2. TRINUCLEOTIDE/NUCLEOTIDE EXPANSION DISEASES

	Expansion	Diseases	Genetics/Radiology
1.	CAG repeats	PolyQ diseases: Mnemonic: SHHADs **S** = SBMA (Kennedy disease) **H** = Huntington's disease **H** = Huntington's-like disease **A** = Ataxias (SCAs) **D** = DRPLA	CAG repeat SCAs • SCA 1,2,3 • SCA 6,7,8 • SCA 12,17
2.	Juvenile-onset HD	Juvenile-onset Huntington's disease Onset <20 years CAG repeat number is high: >55 repeats Abnormal allele inherited from **father (in 75%)*** In some cases, the Juvenile HD may start before HD starts in parents* (anticipation) More the number of repeats, earlier is the onset So disease starts in children before it starts in parents In such cases, a positive family history is not elicitable	Genetic analysis: Chromosome 4 Autosomal dominant CAG repeats MRI brain: Bilateral caudate atrophy Boxcar ventricles
3.	GAA repeats	Friederich's ataxia (see previous pages)	Chromosome 9 Frataxin gene Autosomal recessive
4.	CTG repeats	Myotonic dystrophy	
5.	CGG repeats	FXTAS Fragile X-tremor ataxia syndrome • Usual onset after >50 years • Mainly affects males • Females may be affected (15–20% with premutation) Males: >50 years • Anticipation + • Intellectual disability • Usually have >200 repeats (full mutation) Females: Premutation (55–200 CGG repeats) • Less intellectual disability • Have primary ovarian failure • Less severely affected than males	FMR-1 gene X-chromosome
6.	GCN repeats	OPMD: Oculo-pharyngeal muscular dystrophy (PABP-N1) autosomal dominant	

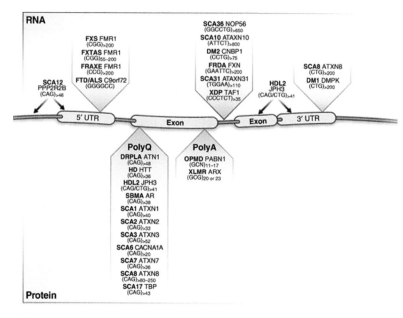

Figure 7.1

3. IMPORTANT GENETIC CONSIDERATIONS IN EPILEPSY

Disease	Clinical	Genetics/Radiology
Carbamazepine (CBZ) in Focal epilepsy	CBZ causes SJS-TEN SJS-TEN: Stevens–Johnson syndrome Risk particularly increased if a person carries the allele FDA recommends testing for it before starting CBZ Especially in ASIAN patients	HLA -B *1502 allele + Studied in Han Chinese

4. PARKINSON'S DISEASE GENETICS

a. 20% Parkinson's are familial.

b. PARK-8 (LRRK2) mutations are the most common cause of both familial and sporadic PD.

c. Autosomal dominant: PARK-8 (LRRK2).

d. Autosomal recessive
   i.   PARK-2 (parkin).
   ii. PARK-6 (PTEN).
   iii. PARK-7 (DJ-1).
   iv. PARK-9 (ATP13a2).

5. GENETICS IN OTHER DEGENERATIVE DISEASES

	Disease	Clinical and pathological features	Genetics/Radiology
1.	**ALS/MND**	ALS is commonly sporadic, but in some cases, ALS may be genetic Biopsy in 97% cases of ALS/MND show • Neuronal and glial inclusions • Biopsy positive for ubiquitin and TDP-43	Sporadic or other ALS SOD-1 mutation positive

	Disease	Clinical and pathological features	Genetics/Radiology
		3% cases are positive for ubiquitin Absent TDP-43 (TAR DNA binding protein 43) **Absence of TDP-43** distinguishes sporadic ALS from **SOD-1 positive genetic ALS**	SOD-1 mutation positive
	MND-FTD	Most common cause of FTD-MND overlap syndrome (Fronto-temporal Dementia—with MND)	C9orf 72 mutation
2.	HNA Hereditary neuralgic amyotrophy	Recurrent branchial plexopathy • Severe pain • Weakness of Upper Limb • Sensory disturbances seen • Symptoms may improve over time or may recur in same limb or the other limb • Family history may be + Other C/P • **Hyper-telorism** (Inter-Pupillary Diameter) • Cleft palate • Skin folds in neck, back, shoulder	Genetics: SEPT-9 gene Figure 7.2
3.	Prion diseases	Prion diseases are transmissible, untreatable and fatal diseases of mammals. There are different kinds of prion diseases like • Genetic prion diseases • Idiopathic • Creutzfeldt–Jakob disease (CJD) • Variant Creutzfeldt–Jakob disease (vCJD) • Gerstmann–Straussler–Scheinker syndrome [a] Fatal Familial Insomnia • Kuru	Genetics PRPN = prion protein gene Polymorphisms @ codon 129 (methionine or valine) 6 isoforms exist MM1 MM2 MV1 MV2 VV1 VV2 Codon 129
4.	Heidenhain variant CJD	This is a peculiar clinical presentation of sporadic CJD There is predominantly occipital involvement Examination is remarkable for presence of Ophthalmic signs—so patients initially go to eye specialist	**MM-1** genotype

6. MISCELLANEOUS GENES IMPORTANT IN NEUROLOGY

	Gene	Description	Disorder
1.	PHYH	Phytanoyl-CoA-hydroxylase Peroxisomal Alpha-oxidation enzyme	Involved in • Phytanic acid metabolism • Refsum disease
2.	GJB-1	Gap-junction-beta-1 Connexin-32	Mutation cause • CMT1x
3.	MPO	Myeloperoxidase Chromosome 17	Alzheimer's dementia

NEURO-ENDOCRINOLOGY AND NEURO-TOXICOLOGY

Abbreviations

- *C/P*: Clinical presentation
- *O/E*: On examination
- *D/D*: Differential diagnosis

Very important clues in any question:

- Any Question with history of **bariatric surgery + vomiting** = Wernicke encephalopathy
- Any Question with history of **bariatric surgery + myeloneuropathy** = Copper deficiency
- Any Question with **Asian heritage** and weakness = Thyroid diseases

1. NUTRITIONAL DISORDERS OF THE NERVOUS SYSTEM

	Condition	Clinical features	Radiology and diagnosis
1.	WE Wernicke encephalopathy	Pathogenesis: Due to Thiamine deficiency Risk factors • Alcoholic person • **Bariatric** surgery** • Gastric bypass surgery • Malnutrition • Pregnancy MC C/P: **Vomiting**** • No fever • O/E: Ophthalmoplegia • Gait ataxia Investigations: Routine bloods normal Triad of (C-O-G): • Alteration in **C**onsciousness • **O**cular dysfunction • **G**ait abnormalities Classic **triad is seen in only 20–40**% cases Most patients present with 2 out of 3 features	Symmetric lesions in • Thalamus • III ventricle: Periventricular • Peri-aqueduct area • Mamillary bodies • Tectal plate • Peri-acqueductal grey **Alcoholics**: Contrast enhancement of **thalamus and MB**** Non-alcoholics: Atypical findings common: Hyperintensities seen in • Cerebellum • Cranial nerve nuclei D/D: Metronidazole-induced cerebral damage: MRI—same areas affected Rx: Intravenous thiamine

(Continued)

DOI: 10.1201/b23306-8

(Continued)

	Condition	Clinical features	Radiology and diagnosis
1.	WE Wernicke encephalopathy (Contd)	Figure 8.1 MRI brain T2/FLAIR in a patient of Wernicke Encephalopathy: Showing hyperintensities around the III ventricle in mid-brain and in bilateral thalamus	

Similar lesions can be seen in MIE, but the classical lesions of MIE also include lesions in the Dentate nucleus and in splenium of corpus callosum.

	Condition	Clinical features	Radiology and diagnosis
2.	MIE Metronidazole-induced encephalopathy	Rare side effect of metronidazole Dysarthria Gait ataxia Nystagmus • Horizontal nystagmus in both directions • Lesions reverse after stopping metronidazole	MRI brain: Lesions are due to vasogenic edema Bilateral + symmetrical lesions seen in • Dentate Nucleus *** • Midbrain • Dorsal pons • Dorsal medulla Lesions of splenium of Corpus callosum are not due to edema
3.	Celiac disease	Cause: Gluten sensitivity • C/P with ataxia • Nystagmus • Absent reflexes • Sensory loss • Sensori-motor axonopathy	2 in 3 patients will have cerebellar atrophy (MRI) Genetics: Association with HLA Dq2, DQ8
		Most common C/P of celiac disease: Gluten enteropathy. Only a small number of patients with gluten ataxia will have concomitant GIT symptoms Only **1 in 3** will have biopsy-proven enteropathy 2 in 3 patients will have cerebellar atrophy	
4.	Copper deficiency	Copper deficiency can cause myeloneuropathy It is a treatable cause of Non-compressive Myelopathy C/P like SACD of B12 deficiency Posterior column involvement—ataxia	Serum copper level: <0.1 mcg/mL MRI abnormalities in 50%: • High T2 signal in posterior column of spine • Long segment involvement—post-cervical + thoracic cord

	Condition	Clinical features	Radiology and diagnosis
		Sensory ataxia + absent reflexes. Motor neuropathy may co-exist	Hallmark is CBC and peripheral smear findings.
		Clues in Question to diagnose copper deficiency myeloneuropathy: <ul><li>History of Upper GI surgery</li><li>Bariatric surgery</li><li>Malabsorption syndrome</li><li>**intake of ZINC!!**</li><li>**Microcytic anemia +**</li><li>**Leucopenia ** **</li><li>May also have normocytic or macrocytic anemia</li></ul>	

2. STORAGE DISEASES

	Condition	Clinical features	Radiology and diagnosis
1.	NP-C Niemann-Pick disease–type C	Heterogenous disorder Autosomal recessive inheritance Variable presentation Can present anytime: from Perinatal-to-adulthood <ul><li>Psychiatric features +</li><li>Hepatomegaly in 50% +</li><li>Splenomegaly in 90% +</li><li>Vertical gaze palsy +</li><li>Cerebellar ataxia +</li><li>Parkinsonism</li><li>Cognitive and executive abnormalities</li><li>Perceptive deafness</li></ul>	NPC1 gene mutation + Filipin staining of fibroblast cell culture Clinical features which can present at any age <ul><li>Gaze palsy</li><li>Hearing problems</li><li>Ataxia</li><li>Parkinsonian symptoms</li><li>SPLEEENNNNNomegaly</li></ul>
2.	Gaucher disease	Liposomal disorder Mutation in GBA1 Pathogenesis: Dysfunction of beta-gluco-cerebrosidase enzyme Leads to accumulation of glucocerebroside (sphingolipid) in cells and tissues C/P: Same as NP-C <ul><li>Usually 20–40 years</li><li>Psychiatric symptoms ++</li><li>Hepatomegaly 50%,</li><li>splenomegaly 90%</li><li>parkinsonism</li></ul>	Diagnostic clues <ul><li>Eyes: Yellow spots</li><li>Anemia, thrombocytopenia in 90%</li><li>Bone pains, joint pains</li><li>Growth retardation, easy bruising, bleeding</li></ul> Diagnosis is made by: a. Decreased enzyme levels b. Increased in ALP c. Biopsy findings d. Genetic testing
3.	KRS Kufor–Rakeb syndrome	Inherited disorder Parkinson- 9 Juvenile-onset Parkinson (teenagers) C/P: Similar to NPC <ul><li>Autosomal recessive</li><li>**Supranuclear gaze** palsy</li><li>Spasticity may be +</li></ul>	MRI shows: Nigro-straiatal-pallidal-pyramidal degeneration ATP13A2 mutation Classical feature is a supranuclear palsy

3. ENDOCRINOLOGICAL DISORDERS AFFECTING THE NERVOUS SYSTEM

	Condition	Clinical features	Radiology and diagnosis
1.	TPP Thyrotoxic periodic paralysis	Characterized by Attacks of weakness similar to hypoKalemic periodic paralysis More common in ASIANS!!** • Proximal weakness + areflexia • Bulbar functions are normal • Respiratory normal Prior history of • Heavy meals or • Exercise before onset of weakness	Lab tests: **Hypokalemia**∗∗ Clues in question to identify TPP • Asian person • Graves' disease • **Weight loss** • **Diarrhea** • **Palpitations** • High T3 T4 levels • Weakness settles with normalization of thyroid
		The differential diagnosis of acute-onset areflexic quadriparesis can be • Hypokalemic periodic paralysis • Thyrotoxic periodic paralysis • GBS—will have bulbar and respiratory weakness also	
2.	Myxedema coma	Myxedema coma is a life-threatening emergency The main clinical presentation is: • Mental status changes + 4 Hypo's • HYPOthermia • HYPOtension, Bradycardia • HYPOglycemia • HYPO- or areflexia • Non-pitting edema face, arms, legs • Periorbital swelling • Generalized puffiness • MACROGLOSSIA, PTOSIS	Clues in question • Feeling COLD • Everything is HYPO, except • Tongue—macroglossia • Swelling—edema Rx • Thyroid replacement + hydrocortisone • Unless adrenal insufficiency is ruled out • Failure to Rx with steroids will precipitate adrenal crisis
3.	Addison crisis	C/P • Hyponatremia • Weight loss • Dehydration • Muscle wasting • Loss of sex hormone—amenorrhea	• Hyperkalemia • Hypercalcemia • Hyperpigmentation • High renin • High ACTH
4.	AIP/PRES	AIP = Acute intermittent porphyria PRES = Posterior reversible encephalopathy syndrome PRES in setting of abdominal pain and CNS deficits: Always suspect AIP Clinical features: • Autosomal dominant disease • Severe abdominal colic • Psychiatric symptoms • Autonomic symptoms • Neurological deficits • Nausea, vomiting, diarrhea • Confusion • Muscle weakness + numbness Attacks are precipitated by • Alcohol • Any Illness • Medication (OCP, sulpha drugs) • Menstruation	Blood tests: Deficiency of Porphobilinogen deaminase (hydroxymethybilane) This leads to: Accumulation of porphobilinogen In cytoplasm Investigation: 24-**hour urine porphobilinogen**∗∗ increased 6Ps • Porphobilinogen deficiency • Pain abdomen • Psychiatric symptoms • Peripheral neuropathy • Pee abnormalities (dysuria) • Precipitated by drugs Rx: High-Carbohydrate diet + supplements; IV glucose + haem like substances

4. TOXIC DISEASES

		Clinical features and pathogenesis	Clues and diagnosis
1.	Lead toxicity	Inhalation of inorganic lead in form of • Fumes, mist, vapours • Wall paint • From Georgian buildings • Electrical works Clinically, lead toxicity presents with **Pure motor** neuropathy • Radial nerve • Peroneal nerve, causing Weakness of wrist extension, finger extension, wrist drop, finger drop	**A**: Anemia (microcytic) **B**: Basophilic strippling **C**: Colicky pain **D**: Diarrhea/constipation **E**: Encephalopathy (rare) **F**: Facial pallor (earliest)** **G**: Gum lines (Burtonian) **H**: Hormonal problems Blood lead levels: >25 mcg/dL MRI: Bilateral **thalami and lentiform** hyperintensity Rx: EDTA, DMSA, meso-2,3-dimercaptosucc
2.	Ciguatera toxin	Ciguatera is a seafood, reef fish **Most common toxicity associated with seafood** Acute poisoning leads to • P: Parastheshia/perioral numbness • P: Painful micturition • A: Autonomic dysfunction • D: Dysesthesia, diarrhea • H: Headache • GIT symptoms Chronic poisoning leads to fatigue Chronic fatigue syndrome**	Clinical presentation mnemonic: PADH-tummy

3.	TCA drugs
	 Tricyclic antidepressants
	 Amitriptyline
	 Nortriptyline
		TCA toxicity will present with
		 • Drowsiness
		 • Confusion
		 • Seizures or coma
		 • Anticholinergic side effects like
		    • Dry mouth
		    • Blurred vision
		    • No sweating
		    • High body temperature— can't dissipate heat
		    • Tachycardia
		    • Hypotension
			Clues in Question
			 • Background migraine
			 • Depression
			 • Hyperthermia
			 • ECG: Prolonged QT arrythmias/tachycardia

4.	SS Serotonin syndrome	Recent Parkinson's disease patient started on serotonin drugs and has the following clinical features • **Sweaty**!! + 3H-TR • **H**yperthermia • **H**ypertension • **H**yperreflexic • **T**achycardia • Somnolent/Altered sensorium/ Delirium	Drugs causing SS: When you START taking these drugs or DOSE of these drugs is increased • MAO inhibitors • SSRI drugs • Triptans • SNRI, TCA • Buspirone • Metoclopramide, ondansetrone

(Continued)

(Continued)

		Clinical features and pathogenesis	Clues and diagnosis
		D/D: Neuroleptic malignant syndrome–SS has abrupt onset + **normal labs + clonus**	• St John's wort, Cocaine • Antiepileptics: Valproate • CBZ, oxcarbazepine • Opioids—buprenorpine, tramadol

	Serotonin syndrome	Neuroleptic malignant syndrome
Drugs causing	Serotonergic drugs	Dopamine antagonists
Examination reveals	Hyperreflexia Clonus Myoclonus Ocular clonus	More rigidity Leads pipe rigidity Hyporeflexia High temperature
Laboratory tests	Usually normal	High CPK (creatine kinase) High WBC count Low serum iron
Course of illness	Fast onset Starts within 1–2 days of starting the drug	Slow onset Takes 1–2 weeks to start after introducing the drug
Resolves within	Few days	10–14 days

5.	OP
	Organophosphate poisoning
		• Altered sensorium +
		• Increased secretions +
		• **Bradycardia + SWEATY**!!
		• All secretions are increased: DUMBELLS
		  D = Diarrhea
		  U = Increased urination
		  M = Miosis
		  B = Bronchial secretions
		  E = Emesis
		  L = Lacrimation
		  S = Sweating
			Intermediate syndrome less common with Carbamates
			More common with OP

		In next 4 days: Patients may develop intermediate syndrome characterized by • Neck flexion weakness • Proximal weakness • Absent reflexes • Bilateral facial weakness • Motor cranial nerve weakness • Respiratory weakness	
6.	Platinum compounds Cisplatin	Cisplatin is used in DHAP regimen for Hodgkin's lymphoma Cisplatin toxicity causes • Non-length dependent neuropathy • **Sensory ganglionopathy** • Absent reflexes • Gait ataxia • Sensory loss in **FACE, hands** and feet	Nerve conduction studies: Absent SNAPs **Normal CMAPs**!! SNAP: Sensory nerve action potential CMAP: Compound muscle action potential

		Clinical features and pathogenesis	Clues and diagnosis
7.	Vitamin B6 toxicity	Pyridoxine overdose causes Sensory ganglionopathy Vitamin B6 supplements are commonly given in tuberculosis patients, who are taking Isoniazid	In patients on anti-tubercular therapy, not giving Pyridoxine can lead to isoniazid-induced neuropathy Conversely, excess of Pyridoxine can also cause sensory ganglionopathy
8.	Methanol toxicity	Risk factors • Homemade liquor • Local-made liquor • Improper distillation C/P • Blindness • Optic atrophy	 Figure 8.2 MRI brain: Putaminal necrosis in methanol toxicity.
		Putaminal necrosis: Seen in **CO.C.E.M.**** • **CO: Carbon monoxide** • **Cyanide,** • **Ethylene glycol** and • **Methanol** If Optic atrophy is present, it is more suggestive of Methanol toxicity	

5. NEURO-OTOLOGY

	Maneuver/Test/Procedure	Explanation	Special points
1.	Dix–Hallpike Maneuver	Positional test Gold standard test to diagnose BPPV Used in diagnosis of • Posterior canal BPPV	Sensitivity for Posterior canal BPPV = 90%
2.	Epley's maneuver	Used in the treatment of • Posterior canal BPPV	
3.	Brandt–Daroff exercises	Used in treatment of • Posterior canalithiasis	
4.	Cawthorne–Cooksey exercises	Used in treatment of • Posterior canal BPPV	
5.	Anterior/superior canal BPPV	Diagnosis: Supine head hanging test	Treatment • Reverse Epley maneuver • Yacovino maneuvers • Short CRP: Canalith repositioning maneuvers
6.	Horizontal/Lateral canal BPPV	Diagnosis: Supine roll test	Treatment: Gufoni maneuver

(Continued)

(Continued)

	Maneuver/Test/ Procedure	Explanation	Special points
7.	PST/TT Paroxysmal staccato tinnitus/typewriter tinnitus	Sound of typewriter or machine gun Or morse code Daily transient attacks Lasting 10–15 seconds Increased by head turning or loud noise Associated nausea, vomiting, vertigo may be present Cause: Neuro-vascular compression of VIII nerve; though low sensitivity	This comes under a spectrum of diseases; including VP/TT Rx: Respond very well to Carbamazepine Response to carbamazepine is almost diagnostic for PST/TT
8.	VP Vestibular paroxysmia	This comes under a spectrum of diseases, including VP/TT	In VP: Vertigo is the main C/P In TT: Tinnitus is the main C/P
9.	MdDS Mal de debarquement syndrome Disembarkement syndrome	Subjective feeling of motion @ rest Feeling of swaying or rocking Impaired cognition Kinesiophobia Risk Factor: Prolonged exposure to motion • Roller coaster rides, seasickness, air travel, motion games	Rx • SSRI • BZD benzodiazepines
10.	PLF Perilymph fistula	Connection between the inner ear perilymph and air-filled space of middle ear Results in Perilymph leaking into the middle ear Caused by trauma • Barotrauma • Head trauma • CSOM • Valsalva C/P: Same ear hearing loss • Ongoing dizziness • No cerebellar signs	**Fistula test** Press on the tragus Apply +/– pressure on intact TM (tympanic membrane) Onset of nystagmus or disequilibrium means positive fistula test
11.	Mèniére's disease (MD)	Triad Vertigo + tinnitus + aural fullness With or w/o hearing loss There is an overlap of symptoms between MD and VM: Vestibular migraine In VM: There is history of migraine + • Headache • Photophobia, phono • Aura In MD: Documented hearing loss during or after attack	**D/D: VP: Hypoacusis**
	In an Emergency room: When a patient comes with sudden-onset giddiness		
12.	Sudden-onset giddiness, ataxia and vertigo may be due to ear disorder or due to cerebellar causes Ataxic gait may be central or peripheral pathology Check vestibular reflexes Do HINTS test; See nystagmus Right beating nystagmus = right cerebellum lesion or Or left vestibular lesion		

6. STATISTICS: SOME IMPORTANT FORMULAE

a. *Calculate relative risk/risk-ratio*

$$\frac{\text{Probability of disease in exposed} \div}{\text{Probability of disease in non-exposed}}$$

$$\frac{A \div (A+B)}{C \div (C+D)}$$

b. *Calculate odds ratio (OR)*
Odds ratio Quantifies the strength of association between any 2 events

$$OR = \frac{(A \times D)}{(B \times C)}$$

c. NNT = Number needed to treat
NNT = 1/ARR (absolute risk reduction)

How to calculate NNT

   i. Calculate the risk in the treatment arm (risk of death)—e.g., 25%
   ii. Calculate risk in control arm—e.g., 30%
   iii. ARR = 30–25% = 5%
   iv. NNT = 1/ARR = 1/5 = 20

	Disease	Controls
Exposed	A	B
Not exposed	C	D

Figure 8.3

The Truth

Test Score:	Has the disease	Does not have the disease	
Positive	True Positives (TP) a	False Positives (FP) b	$PPV = \dfrac{TP}{TP + FP}$
Negative	c False Negatives (FN)	d True Negatives (TN)	$NPV = \dfrac{TN}{TN + FN}$

Sensitivity	Specificity
$\dfrac{TP}{TP + FN}$	$\dfrac{TN}{TN + FP}$

Or,

$\dfrac{a}{a + c}$	$\dfrac{d}{d + b}$

Figure 8.4   Calculation of sensitivity, specificity, PPV and NPV.

7. ETHICS

Principle	Explanation	
Bolam principle Bolam test	The Bolam test is based on the premise of determining whether the actions of the doctor are in line with the actions of other medics who are in their position (same medical skills) It states that if a doctor reaches the standard of a responsible body of medical opinion, they are not negligent	
	Examples <ul><li>Performing a surgery with or without anesthesia</li><li>Giving ECT for mental illness without skeletal muscle relaxants</li><li>Performing orthopedic surgeries</li><li>Any new drug/technique gaining popularity</li></ul>	**In all these situations, Bolam principle will help in defense of a doctor as he would act in an acceptable standard of care.**
Gillick competency	Gillick competency is often used to assess whether a child is mature enough to consent to treatment	
	Used in UK and Wales Used for a child to decide the functional ability to make a decision regarding treatment without the need of parent or elderly guidance	For example: **Immunization Surgery for pediatric diseases**
Occam's razor	Simplest explanation is the best explanation	
Hickam's dictum	A patient can have as many diseases as he damn well pleases Counter-argument to Occam's razor in medical science	
Declaration of Geneva	Came out in 1948—one of the oldest Accepted by WHO Physician's dedication to the humanitarian goals of medicine Oath for physicians	
Declaration of Helsinki	Ethical principles regarding human experimentation developed originally in 1964 for the medical community by the World Medical Association (WMA)	

NEURO-INFLAMMATORY DISEASES

Abbreviations

- *ADEM*: Acute disseminated encephalomyelitis
- *CJD*: Creutzfeldt–Jakob disease
- *d/d*: Differential diagnosis
- *MOG*: Myelin oligodendrocyte disorders
- *MS*: Multiple sclerosis
- *NMO*: Neuromyelitis optica
- *SPS*: Stiff person syndrome

1. CNS INFLAMMATORY DISORDERS AND AUTOIMMUNE ENCEPHALITIS

	Disease	Clinical features	Diagnosis and management
1.	ADEM Acute disseminated encephalomyelitis	Uncommon disease • Widespread inflammation and demyelination in CNS • Brain and spinal cord involvement • 2 types of ADEM are known • Post-infectious ADEM • Post-vaccinal ADEM	MRI: Confluent T2 hyperintensities; enhancing supra-tentorial lesions + Thalamus, brainstem and Spinal cord involvement CSF: Pleocytosis High CSF protein levels
2.	Anti-NMDA-receptor encephalitis	It is a common autoimmune encephalitis Also reported to occur after herpes simplex encephalitis. C/P: There are 5 stages described in this disorder • Prodromal stage • Psychotic stage: Neuro-psychiatric syndrome • Unresponsive stage • Hyperkinetic stage • Gradual recovery phase	ICU care is very important because of • Recurrent seizures • Dysautonomia • Fluctuating sensorium MRI: <50% cases have T2/flair hyperintensities involving the Frontal and mesial temporal lobes Leptomeningeal enhancement may be seen Serology: Anti-NMDA receptor antibodies positive in serum/CSF

(Continued)

DOI: 10.1201/b23306-9

(Continued)

	Disease	Clinical features	Diagnosis and management
2.	Anti-NMDA-receptor encephalitis (Contd)	Common clinical manifestations include: • Agitation, and hallucinations • Psychiatric and behavior changes occur @ onset • Various abnormal movements • Orofacial dyskinesia, chorea, athetosis, dystonia • Myorrhythmia, ophisthotonus • Ballismus, blepharospasm, oculo gyric crisis	Rx: IVIG, Rituximab Anti-NMDA encephalitis is also reported with OVARIAN TERATOMA Prognosis is good in 80%
3.	MFS Miller Fisher Syndrome	One of the rare forms of a demyelinating disease. It is included in the spectrum of Guillain–Barré syndrome MFS is a triad of • Ataxia: Broad-based ataxic gait • Areflexia • Ophthalmoparesis Pathogenesis of GBS/MFS: • Molecular mimicry	**Serology: GQ1b antibodies are seen in 80–95%** GQ1b antibody has a postulated role in pathogenesis of **ophthalmoplegia** CSF: Albumino-Cytological Dissociation (~GBS) NCS: Absent H reflex, reduced SNAPs (~GBS) Rx: IVIG, Plasmapheresis
4.	BBE Bickerstaff brainstem encephalitis	BBE is also classified in the spectrum of Guillain–Barré syndrome Pathogenesis: • Post-infectious: Viral infection • Molecular mimicry C/P • Mostly central/brainstem-related manifestations • Altered sensorium • Ophthalmoplegia • Hyperreflexia • Symmetric flaccid quadriplegia may develop	GQ1b antibody positive in 66% cases MRI is usually normal MRI may be abnormal in 33% cases Rx: IVIG, Plasmapheresis

5.	CLIPPERS
	Chronic lymphocytic inflammation with pontocerebellar perivascular enhancement responsive to steroids
		Described by Pittock et al. in 2011
		CLIPPERS is a rare form of CNS inflammatory disease D/D: CLIPPERS
		• Glioma
		• Large B-cell lymphoma
		• CNS angiitis
		
		Pathogenesis of CLIPPERS is still not elucidated
			CLIPPERS has a characteristic imaging appearance:
			• MRI: Punctate and curvilinear hyperintensities in brainstem:
			  • Peppering of pons
			  • Extending into Midbrain and cerebellum
			
			Biopsy: CD3 and some CD 20 Lymphocytic infiltrate in White matter; In perivascular spaces
			
			Treatment is with steroids

	Disease	Clinical features	Diagnosis and management
6.	SREAT Steroid-responsive encephalopathy associated with autoimmune thyroiditis Hashimoto encephalopathy	Autoimmune encephalopathy Autoimmune condition characterized by elevated thyroid autoantibodies with cognitive dysfunction; responsive to corticosteroids 2 types of clinical presentations are known a. Recurrent stroke and acute and sub-acute progression b. Chronic progression with • Encephalopathy • Myoclonus • Tremors • Hallucinations • Dysphasia • Seizures • Gait ataxia	Sometimes it is a diagnosis of exclusion Serum: Anti-TPO antibody and anti-TG antibody positive High ALT levels CSF: High protein levels Very common d/d • CJD • Dementia • Viral encephalitis
7.	PERM (SPS-plus) Progressive encephalo-myelitis with rigidity and myoclonus	Severe syndrome that presents with • Autonomic features • Hyperekplexia (brainstem myoclonus) • Painful spasms • Breathing problems Common and classical features include: Spontaneous and stimulus sensitive myoclonus **Axial rigidity** Painful spasms ~ SPS Brainstem dysfunction **Autonomic dysfunction** • Profuse sweating • Urinary retention, tachycardia Sometimes spasms and rigidity are so severe that they may result in fractures	Serology: GAD antibody positive Rx: Immune therapy • Steroids • Rituximab • IVIG There are rare case reports of post-infectious PERM (e.g. after brucellosis)
8.	Anti-DPPX (K channel)	Resembles PERM But has a prodrome of diarrhea/gastric symptoms So, patient has diarrhea followed by progressive CNS features • Cognitive decline • Hyperexcitability	Serology DPPX antibodies positive Rx: Immunotherapy

2. PARANEOPLASTIC ENCEPHALITIS SYNDROMES

	Disease	Clinical features	Diagnosis and management
1.	OMS Opsoclonus myoclonus syndrome OMAS Opsoclonus myoclonus ataxia syndrome	Also called • Dancing Eyes–Dancing Feet Syndrome • Kinsbourne syndrome A rare autoimmune/paraneoplastic condition that usually affects young children Mean age of diagnosis: 18–24 months C/P • Ataxia • Imbalance • Opsoclonus: Eyes—Haphazard extraocular movements in all directions • Myoclonus	Most common associations • Neuroblastoma • **Small cell lung cancer*** Para-infectious OMS has been reported with • Viral illness • Lyme disease • Chikungunya fever
2.	Anti-**Tr** Antibodies encephalitis	Paraneoplastic cerebellar degeneration (PCD)	Associated with **HODGKIN'S** lymphoma
3.	Anti-Amphiphysin antibody encephalitis	Causes paraneoplastic SPS • Rigidity • Hyper-lordosis • Weight loss	Most common association • **Breast cancer***
4.	Anti-GABA-A antibody encephalitis	Autoimmune/paraneoplastic encephalitis characterized by • Encephalitis + **Seizures**** • Status epilepticus • Cognitive impairment • Loss of consciousness • Movement disorders Commonly presents with Status epilepticus	MRI brain: Gray matter + White Matter abnormality in frontal and temporal lobes CSF: Abnormal in 50% cases High cell and protein Associated with • **Thymoma**** • Viral infections • Autoimmune disorders
5.	Kelch-like protein 11-associated encephalitis	KLHL-11 PNS: Kelch-like protein 11-associated paraneoplastic neurological disorder C/P • Hearing loss** • Rhombencephalitis—ataxia • Limbic encephalitis • Opsoclonus myoclonus syndrome	Serology • HLA DQB 1*02 • HLA DRB 1*03 Associated with • **Testicular seminoma*** • **Ovarian tumours**

	Disease	Clinical features	Diagnosis and management
6.	Carcinomatous meningitis	Dissemination of malignant cells from primary tumour sites to leptomeningeal layers • Occurs in the advanced stage of • Solid as well as hematological cancers • Rare complication • Very poor prognosis. Presentation is similar to any meningitis, but high degree of suspicion is required for diagnosis.	Most common cause: • Breast cancer >> Lung cancer CSF analysis should be done to look for malignant cells with cytospin technology
7.	Anti-Hu antibody paraneoplastic syndrome	Mainly presents as Sensory ganglionopathy In association with tumours/lung cancer • Impaired Joint position and vibration • Pseudo-athetosis • Absent deep tendon reflexes	**Lung** cancer** NCS: Symmetrical, non-length dependent sensory neuropathy Non-recordable sensory amplitudes

3. IMMUNE-MEDIATED NEUROMUSCULAR DISORDERS

1.	MMN-CB Multifocal motor neuropathy with conduction blocks	MMN-CB is a rare, acquired, motor neuropathy Common clinical features are: • Affects males <50 years Males >> Females Upper limb onset • Wrist drop/finger drop/foot drop • Sensory grossly normal Purely motor involvement: In the distribution of single nerve—but without sensory involvement	Serology: Anti-GM1 antibodies + Rx: Robust response to immune therapy: IVIG Because of predominant and asymmetric motor involvement, it can mimic MND (motor neuron disease) Compared to MMN-CB, CIDP is a more symmetrical and diffuse disease
2.	MG Myasthenia gravis	Chronic autoimmune disorder of the neuromuscular junction • Fatiguable weakness • Mostly, starts in the eyes with • Ptosis, ophthalmoplegia • Pure motor weakness • May cause respiratory and bulbar weakness Autoimmune antibodies • Anti-acetylcholine receptor antibodies (ACh-R) • Muscle-specific kinase antibodies: MuSK • Anti-LRP4 • Agrin antibodies	Most common antibody: ACh-R False-positive Ach-R antibodies may be seen in • Rheumatoid arthritis • Penicillamine intake ACh-R positivity has high specificity for MG (99% specific) ACh-R negativity has high specificity for absent thymoma Ocular Myasthenia: ACh-R in **70**% cases of ocular myasthenia MUSK positivity means chances of thymoma are <1%

(Continued)

(Continued)

		Thymoma: Seen in some cases of myasthenia • Has been reported to be pathogenic in myasthenia • Recurrence of thymoma seen in 10–30% patients after surgery • Always search for thymoma in any patient of MG • Always search for thymoma if patient has refractory symptoms despite thymoma resection and med management Use of Steroids: Always remember • Steroid use can usually increase the total cell count in blood • TLC in patients of steroids may be between 15,000–17,000/mm • Don't misdiagnose these patients as having infection (can see ESR, CRP levels)	
3.	ICI-MG	**Immune check point** inhibitor–induced myasthenia Due to the use of • CTLA-4 or PD I-1 inhibitor drugs: **Nevolimab** • These drugs are used in renal cell carcinoma (RCC) and other cancers C/P: Similar to any myasthenic syndrome • Eyes: Ptosis, ophthalmoplegia • Proximal muscle weakness • Head drop, dysarthria • Proximal myopathy/**myositis** • Mean serum CPK levels 2500–3000 Other manifestations • Myocarditis • Hepatitis • Colitis • Thyroiditis • AIHA: Autoimmune hemolytic anemia	
4.	LEMS Lambert–Easton myasthenia syndrome	Autoimmune neuromuscular junction disorder similar to myasthenia However, LEMS is a pre-ganglionic disorder as compared to MG which is a post-ganglionic disorder Proximal weakness + areflexia + Autonomic **Dry mouth**** > ED and constipation Ptosis develops during course (not @ onset)** Autoimmune antibodies **90% LEMS have VGCC** (specificity 99%) 60% LEMS have SOX-1 30% LEMS have anti-Hu	50% LEMS have tumours 90% will have Small Cell Lung cancer (SCLC) @ 3 months 95% will have SCLC @ 1 year High-frequency (50 Hz) RNS and post-exercise stimulation: Shows increase in CMAP >100% Rx • 3,4 AMP • Steroids • AZA: Azathioprine
5.	Paraneoplastic LEMS	C/P • Proximal myopathy • Cerebellar ataxia (10% LEMS) • Ataxia predicts presence of cancer	**Most common tumour: SCLC***

| 6. | Bing–Neel syndrome** | Rare disease
Complication of Waldenström's macroglobulinemia (WM)
Cause
<ul><li>CNS involvement by malignant cells</li><li>Infiltration of the central nervous system by malignant lymphoplasmacytic cells</li></ul>C/P
<ul><li>Manifests few months to years after WM</li><li>Ataxia + cranial nerve palsies is the most common C/P</li><li>Facial palsy</li><li>Ptosis</li><li>Sensory abnormalities</li><li>DTR: Absent reflexes</li></ul> | CSF: High protein in CSF
CSF can also show:
Lympho-plasmacytoid cells

MRI brain: Peri-ventricular and sub-cortical hyperintensities and leptomeningeal enhance
Spinal cord involvement is uncommon

Prognosis: Poor
Mean survival: 4–6 years |

4. MULTIPLE SCLEROSIS (MS) DIAGNOSTIC CRITERIA

Clinical attacks	Radiological lesions	Additional data needed
≥ 2	≥2	None
	1*	
	1	DIS—lesions due to additional clinical attack in a different CNS site or a different MRI lesion
1	≥2	DIT—additional clinical attack Or CSF oligoclonal bands
	1	DIS—lesions due to additional clinical attack in a different CNS site or a different MRI lesion (and) DIT—additional clinical attack Or CSF oligoclonal bands

Source: 2017 modification of the McDonald criteria: Thompson et al, *Lancet Neurology*.

a. DIS: Dissemination in space: Lesions in 2 of 4 locations
   i. Periventricular: PV.
   ii. Juxta cortical: JC.
   iii. Infratentorial.
   iv. Spinal cord: SC.
b. DIT: Dissemination in time
   i. Enhancing + Non-Enhancing lesions on MRI.
   ii. CSF DIT: Oligoclonal bands (OCB)
c. CSF IgG patterns
   i. Pattern III: Identical OCB in serum and CSF with extra in CSF = intrathecal + systemic IgG synthesis—Most important.
   ii. Pattern II: Bands in CSF only = intrathecal only.
   iii. Pattern IV: Bands in both serum and CSF = systemic only.
   iv. Pattern V: Ladder type pattern: Monoclonal peripheral synthesis.
   v. One band in CSF = Monoclonal band—rarely seen in MS.

5. LESIONS IN CNS DEMYELINATION DISORDERS

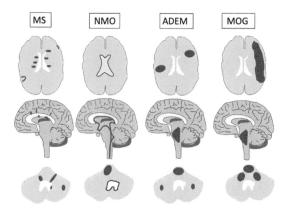

Figure 9.1

	NMO	MOG
	Neuro-myelitis optica syndrome	Myelin-Oligo-dendrocyte-associated disease
Sex	More common in females	Males = females
Eye involvement	Figure 9.2 Schematic representation of optic nerve involvement in NMO (on the left: chiasmal segment) and in MOG (on the right: more anterior involvement).	
Course of illness	Recurrent attacks High relapse rates	Monophasic course more common Less relapse rates
Site of involvement	Cervical and thoracic spine more common	Conus involvement more common
Disability	More severe Poor visual outcomes	Less severe Better visual outcomes
In children	Less common	Can present as ADEM/Encephalopathy

NEURORADIOLOGY AND NEUROPATHOLOGY

Abbreviations

- *EDH*: Extradural hemorrhage
- *ICH*: Intracranial hemorrhage
- *SAH*: Sub-arachnoid hemorrhage
- *SDH*: Subdural hemorrhage

1. BASICS OF CT AND MRI

<table>
<tr><td colspan="3" align="center">CT and MRI sequences</td></tr>
<tr>
<td>NCCT head</td>
<td>Non-contrast CT scan of head
Best for identifying
• Bleeds (EDH, SDH, ICH, SAH)
• Fractures, trauma
• Calcifications</td>
<td>NCCT in SAH
100% sensitive for SAH within 6 hours</td>
</tr>
<tr>
<td>MRI-STIR
Short tau inversion recovery</td>
<td>(T1 inversion)
• Highly water sensitive
• Suppress fat

Combination of T1 and STIR is used to compare fat and water in a body part</td>
<td>Water is white on STIR</td>
</tr>
<tr>
<td>MRI DWI/ADC</td>
<td>DWI—diffusion weighted sequence
ADC—apparent diffusion coefficient

Best sequence for identifying acute infarct
Acute infarct is earliest identified on DWI/ADC</td>
<td>Cytotoxic edema (like in acute stroke)
• T2 hyperintense
• DWI hyperintense
• ADC hypointense

Vasogenic edema appears
• Hyperintense on T2
• Hypointense DWI
• Hyperintense on ADC</td>
</tr>
<tr>
<td>Hemorrhage</td>
<td colspan="2">The appearance of hemorrhage on MRI sequences can indicate the age of bleed

<table>
<tr><th>Age</th><th>Time</th><th>T1</th><th>T2</th></tr>
<tr><td>Hyper-acute</td><td><24 hours</td><td>Iso-intense</td><td>Bright</td></tr>
<tr><td>Acute</td><td>1–3 days</td><td>Iso-intense</td><td>Dark</td></tr>
<tr><td>Early sub-acute</td><td>3–7 days</td><td>Bright</td><td>Dark</td></tr>
<tr><td>Late sub-acute</td><td>7–14 days</td><td>Bright</td><td>Bright</td></tr>
<tr><td>Chronic</td><td>>14 days</td><td>Dark</td><td>Dark</td></tr>
</table>
</td>
</tr>
</table>

(Continued)

(Continued)

Red nucleus	Located in tegmentum of Midbrain Spared in Wilson's disease Forms the enlarged eyes of "GIANT PANDA" 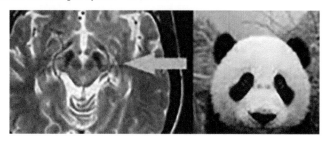 Figure 10.1 Axial T2 MRI in a patient of Wilson's disease.

2. CHIARI MALFORMATION

Types and clinical features	Imaging
Chiari 1: Most common • Seen in females • Descent of cerebellum: Chiari 1 is asymptomatic till adulthood, symptoms depend on degree of descent • Headache (cough headache) and brainstem compression	MRI brain • Pinted tonsils (peg like), • Sulci are vertically oriented • (Sergeant stripes) Crowding of medulla by tonsils in foramen magnum
Chiari 1.5: Descent of cerebellum + brainstem	Draw a line from basion to ophisthion • **<5 mm descent: Benign** low-lying tonsils (ectopia): Not Chiari malformation • Descent 5–10 mm: Asymptomatic, • >12 mm: Usually symptomatic

Associated syndromes
• Klippel–Feil syndrome
• Crouzon syndrome
• Hajdu–Cheney syndromes
	• 30–40% have synringomyelia
	• 30% have hydrocephalus
	• 30–40% have skeletal abnormalities
	  • Platybasia
	  • Invagination
	  • AAO
	  • Sprengel shoulder

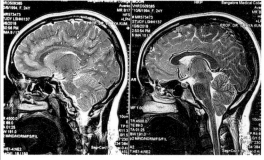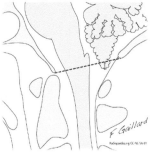

Figure 10.2   Sagittal MRI in a patient with Chiari malformation.

3. NEUROIMAGING IN INFECTIONS

	Infection	Imaging
1.	HIV-related opportunistic infections	(see table below)

Primary CNS Lymphoma	Toxoplasma
Usually single lesion	Multiple lesions
Single + large lesion (>3–4 cm)	Multiple small lesions
More white matter involvement	Basal ganglia
Extensive periventricular involvement	Hemorrhagic lesions
	Multiple ring-enhancing or nodular lesions
Involvement or extension across corpus callosum	"Concentric target" sign
	"Eccentric target" sign

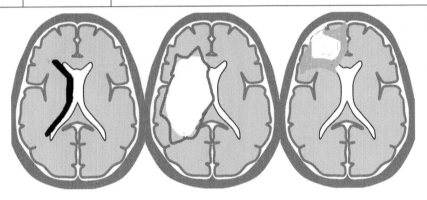

Figure 10.3   Diagrammatic representation of MRI findings in CNS lymphoma.

2.	Intracranial abscess	**DUAL ring** sign in abscess • Hyperintense lesion with • Surrounding vasogenic edema • Outer ring is hypointense • Inner ring is hyperintense • Seen in **75% abscess on T2 and SWI** • There is diffusion restriction in center of abscess • This helps in differentiating from glioblastoma

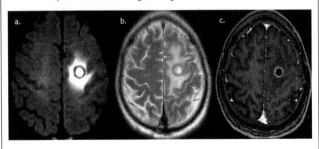

Figure 10.4   Axial MRI (DWI, T2 and T1-contrast) showing left frontal abscess.

(Continued)

(Continued)

	Infection	Imaging
3.	Hydatid cyst (cerebral echinococcosis)	Occurs in 1–2% only Large cystic lesion But small mass effect No perilesional edema The lesion appears • Spherical • Well-defined • Thin-walled **Some contrast enhancement of rim may be seen** C/P: Headache, seizures, focal deficits Figure 10.5 Left frontal hydatid cyst.
4.	CJD Creutzfeldt–Jakob disease	MRI signs in CJD (Creutzfeldt–Jakob disease) • DWI or FLAIR hyperintensities along the cortex • Cortical ribboning • Hockey stick sign in variant CJD Figure 10.6 Axial DWI MRI images showing cortical ribboning in CJD.

4. NEUROIMAGING IN INFLAMMATORY DISEASES

	Disease	Imaging
1.	IIH Idiopathic intracranial hypertension	The most common imaging features are • Flattening of posterior globe** (most specific) • Distention of Optic nerve sheath • Enhancement of pre-laminar Optic nerve • Tortuosity (vertical) of Optic nerve • Empty sella

Figure 10.7   a,b: Empty sella; c,d,e: Thickened, enhancing optic nerve and flattened posterior globe; f: Transverse-sigmoid sinus stenosis.

	Disease	Imaging
2.	SIH Spontaneous intracranial hypotension	**Dural enhancement** **Bilateral symmetrical subdural swelling or SDH** **Venous engorgement, pituitary hyperemia** **Brainstem sagging/slumping which includes** • Ventricular effacement • Effacement of suprasellar and prepontine cistern • Bowing of optic chiasm over sella turcica • Flattening of ventral pons • Downward displacement tonsils Mamillo-pontine distance 5.5 mm or LESS Ponto mesencephalic angle 50 or LESS Both are sensitive and specific for SIH
3.	**CPM/ODS** Central pontine myelinosis/Osmotic demyelination syndrome	**Most common involvement: Ventral pons (basis pontis)**** Cause • CNS damage due to sudden change in osmolality • Secondary to rapid correction of hyponatremia • Extra-pontine myelinosis Other causes of CPM/ODM • Alcohol use • Malnourishment • Diabetes mellitus • Hepatic failure • Cirrhosis • Liver transplant

(Continued)

(Continued)

	Disease	Imaging
3.	**CPM/ODS** Central pontine myelinosis/Osmotic demyelination syndrome (Contd)	MRI • Bilateral signal changes in paramedian pons—T1 hypointense • T2 hyperintense lesions • No contrast enhancement Figure 10.8 Axial MRI showing FLAIR hyperintensities in ventral pons in a patient of CPM.

5. NEUROIMAGING IN NEURODEGENERATION AND POISONINGS

	Condition	Imaging

1.	**FAHR syndrome**
	Idiopathic Basal ganglia calcification
		Bilateral symmetrical basal ganglia calcifications
		
		CT head
		• Calcifications appear hyperdense
		MRI brain
		• Hypointense on GRE/SWI
		• Other metal depositions can also appear hypointense
		    • Calcium
		    • Manganese
		    • Copper
		C/P
		• Can be asymptomatic or may cause subtle symptoms like
		    • Parkinsonism
		    • Headache, seizures
		    • Psychiatric manifestations
		
		Figure 10.9 NCCT head, MRI-T2 and SWI images in a patient of FAHR syndrome.

Differential Diagnosis/Causes of Basal Ganglia Calcification

Degenerative causes	Infectious + metabolic causes	Other causes
• FAHR • PANK mutation • Phenylketonuria 2 • GM1 gangliosidosis • Mitochondrial disease • **Down syndrome** • **Tuberous sclerosis**	• TORCH • Other viruses • Neurocysticercosis • **Hypo-PTH syndrome** • **Pseudo-hypo-PTH** • **Pseudo-pseudo-hypo-PTH** • **Hyper PTH syndrome**	• Lead toxicity • Methotreaxate • Radiation exposure • SLE • VOG malformation • AVM

2.	**NPH** Normal pressure hydrocephalus	Ventricular enlargement disproportionate to cerebral atrophy Evan index >0.3 Callosal angle <90 degree (coronal) Ballooning of frontal horn One or more elliptically dilated sulci Thin and elevation of Corpus callosum Widening of temporal horns CSF flow void in aqueduct Peri-vent hyper intensity—smooth, not CSVD **AC-PC line**: Anterior commissure—posterior commissure line Bi-commissural line Reference plane for axial imaging Callosal angle on coronal imaging is taken perpendicular to AC-PC line

3.	**Progressive
	Supranuclear Palsy**
		MB to pons ratio <0.52 (A/B)
		A <9.35 mm
		Both are 100% specific for PSP
		Named signs on MRI
		   • Hummingbird sign—subjective sign (sagittal)
		   • Mickey Mouse sign (coronal)
		
		Figure 10.10 Sagittal MRI showing the A (midbrain) and B (pons) for calculation of A/B ratio.

(*Continued*)

(Continued)

4.	**MLD** **Metachromatic leukodystrophy**	Autosomal recessive
		MOST COMMON** leukodystrophy
		3 types
		• Infantile onset: 0–3 years
		• Juvenile onset: 3–10 years
		• Adult onset >16 years
		• **Dementia + behavior change + Personality change + Spasticity +**
		• demyelinating sensory motor neuropathy
		• peripheral neuropathy
		• cholecystitis ++
		• MRI: Symmetrical White matter changes—**mainly FRONTAL**
		  • Tigroid pattern
		  • Stripe pattern
		  • Leopard pattern
		  • **Butterfly: Sparing** of sub-cortical U fibres
		• Enzyme: Arylsufatase A deficiency

		Figure 10.11 Schematic representation of findings in A. Alexander disease, B. X-ALD and C. MLD.

5.	**Manganese deposition**	Classical features
		  • T1 hyperintensity in—globus pallidus
		  • Liver cirrhosis
		  • Porto-systemic shunts
		
		Common case scenario
		  • Chronic alcoholic patient
		  • **Poor sensorium**
		  • **Ataxia**
		  • Abdominal distention, ascites, jaundice
		  • High bilirubin, high ALT, low albumin

6.	**CO poisoning** Carbon monoxide	Medial portions of the globus pallidus Areas of low signal intensity on T1-weighted images and High signal intensity on T2-weighted and FLAIR images
		Figure 10.12 Axial T2 and FLAIR MRI images showing bilateral pallidus involvement in CO poisoning.

| 7. | Marchiafava–Bignami | Primary degeneration and atrophy of Corpus callosum (CC)
Demyelination and necrosis of CC
Usually a complication in chronic alcohol consumption
Or malnourishment
Rare disease—has poor outcomes
C/P
   • Altered mental status (confusion)
   • Delirium/loss of consciousness
   • Impaired gait
   • Pyramidal signs
   • Weakness, Rigidity
   • Primitive reflexes
   • Incontinence, GAZE PALSY
   • **CSF normal**
Rx: IV thiamine: Early in course may improve outcome
Outcome better in non-alcoholic group |
| 8. | **Valproate (VPA)–**
induced
hyper-ammonemia | Serious side effect of VPA
Changes in mental status
Focal neurological deficits
Cognitive deficits
Some have increased seizures

MRI: Bilateral basal ganglia hyperintensities
EEG: Diffuse slowing, non-specific
TOPIRAMATE + VPA—increases risk of this
  complication!!**
Rx: Reduce or stop VPA |

6. NEUROIMAGING IN TUMOURS

	Tumour	Imaging

1.	**Pituitary tumours**	Microadenoma <10 mm
		Macroadenoma >10 mm
		All macroadenomas—require surgical management except
		Prolactinomas: Medical management with **Bromocriptine**
		  and cabergoline (Dopamine agonists)
		   • Surgery indicated if hemorrhagic tumour
		   • Progressive visual field deficits (chiasma compression)
		   • No response to medical Rx

2.	**AT**
	Ataxia telangiectasia
		Patients are very sensitive to radiation
		   • Develop cytotoxicity
		   • So avoid at all cost
		   • Even Radiotherapy for cancer in AT be careful
		
		It is preferable to avoid all types of radiotherapy in these
		  patients

3.	**Colloid cyst**	Uncommon tumour
		Always located at roof of IIIrd ventricle
		Adjacent to foramen Monroe
		   • CT head: Appears hyperdense
		   • T1 hyperintense in 50% (maybe iso/hypointense in others)
		   • T2 hypointense usually
		
		Asymptomatic in some cases or may present with acute
		  hydrocephalus

(Continued)

(Continued)

	Tumour	Imaging
4.	**CP angle tumours**	Vestibular schwanommas—most common CP angle tumour—80% CP angle tumours are schwanommas Meningiomas 2nd most common type of CP angle tumour Schwanommas bloom on SWI imaging 100% sensitivity and 92% specificity Because of intra-tumoural hemorrhage in schwanomma—GRE or SWI sequence: Areas of blooming seen

		Vestibular Schwanomma	**Meningioma**
Appearance		Rounded mass in CP angle + internal auditory canal Ice cream cone sign	Sharply demarcated Oval or spherical
		Centered on IAC	Not centered on IAC
NCCT head		Iso- or hypodense No calcification	Hyperdense Calcifications +
CECT		Small tumour: Homogenous enhancement Large tumour: Heterogenous	Bright enhancement

7. NEUROPATHOLOGY

	Disease	Clinical features/Significance	Pathology
1.	IMNM Immune-mediated necrotizing myopathy	Autoimmune necrotizing myopathy Myalgias Proximal weakness + Symmetrical myopathy Dysphagia Highly elevated CPK (>10,000 IU) Resistant to immune-suppressants **Anti-HMGCR** • Anti-3 hydroxy 3 methy-glutary Co reductase • Associated with STATINS intake • Less severe type **Anti-SRP** • More severe type of myopathy	Necrosis ++ No inflammation **There is Myofiber necrosis with lack of inflammation
2.	NFT Neuro-fibrillary tangles	NFT are seen in • Alzheimer's dementia (AD)** • PSP (progressive supranuclear palsy) • Dementia pugilistic • Post-encephalitic Parkinsonism • Guam PD–dementia complex	Difference between NFT and senile plaques • NFT are found inside neurons • Senile plaques outside
	NFT are not seen in: Huntington's chorea		

	Disease	Clinical features/Significance	Pathology
3.	FTD Fronto-temporal dementia	Also called Pick's disease More common in females Predominant behavior and personality changes Frontal executive dysfunction	Biopsy shows Pick bodies: • Which are tangles of abnormal nerve cell proteins called tau proteins.
4.	CBD Cortico-basal degeneration	Sporadic neurodegenerative tauopathy Can have asymmetric symptoms Apraxia Biopsy shows: Ballooned neurons	 Figure 10.13 Ballooned neurons in CBD.
5.	DLBD Dementia with Lewy bodies/Lewy body dementia	Neurodegenerative dementia characterized by abnormal deposits of a protein called alpha-synuclein in the brain Lewy bodies • Pigmented neurons • Abnormal purplish inclusions	 Figure 10.14 Lewy bodies in the nucleus of neuron.
6.	MELAS	Mitochondrial encephalomyopathy, lactic acidosis and stroke-like episodes	Biopsy shows: Ragged red fibres with Gomori trichome stain is the special mitochondrial stain
7.	Tomacula or tomaculous neuropathy	Sausage shape swellings Focal myelin swellings in sural nerve **Seen in** • **HNPP (MC)**** • CIDP • HSMN 1 • HSMN 3 • IgM paraproteinemia	 Figure 10.15 Biopsy findings in Tomaculous neuropathy.
8.	Prions CJD Creutzfeldt–Jakob disease	**Triad of** • **Spongiform vacuolation** • Neuronal loss • Gliosis **Biopsy: Spongiform is the hallmark****	 Figure 10.16 Spongiform vacuolation in CJD.

COGNITIVE DISORDERS AND DEMENTIA

Abbreviations

- *MCI*: Mild cognitive impairment
- *AD*: Alzheimer's dementia
- *FTD*: Fronto-temporal dementia
- *PPA*: Primary progressive aphasia
- *VSNG*: Vertical supranuclear gaze

1. CLINICAL TESTS

Test	Explanation	Scoring
MMSE	Mini-Mental Status Examination MMSE scoring depends on the educational status of the individual	Normal score >24 Maximum score = 30 Dementia if <24
MoCA	Montreal Cognitive Assessment	27–30: Normal score 25–27 = MCI Annual conversion rate to dementia: 10–15%

2. LOCALIZATIONS OF COMMON CLINICAL SIGNS AND SYMPTOMS

	Area	Function and deficits	Disease
1.	Right Temporo-parietal junction	Associated with different capacities that allow to shift attention to unexpected stimuli Also associated with feed-forward and feed-backward information	Presumed to be involved in: Psychogenic or Functional Movement disorders
2.	Left parietal lobe (Dominant inferior parietal lobule)	Dysfunction of dominant inferior parietal lobule causes a tetrad of • Acalculia • Agraphia • Finger agnosia • Right left disorientation	This tetrad is called Gerstman syndrome

(Continued)

DOI: 10.1201/b23306-11

(Continued)

	Area	Function and deficits	Disease
3.	Non-dominant (Right parietal) lobe	Dysfunction of right parietal lobe causes Dressing apraxia Construction apraxia Hemi-spatial sensory neglect Topographical agnosia Anosognosia	
4.	Left anterior temporal lobe	Center of semantic memory (facts) We test it by asking the patient to repeat: • "Pretty-flood-glove-" • "Rough-dough-"	Surface dyslexia Semantic dementia: svPPA(FTD) (semantic variant of PPA)
5.	Anterior thalamic nucleus	Dysfunction causes: • **Anterograde amnesia** with preserved recognition • **Palipsychism**: Superimposition of temporally unrelated information: Interruption of current dialogue with previously discussed unrelated topics	PCA (posterior cerebral artery) stroke: Usually due to tubero- thalamic artery infarction
6.	Left thalamus	Involved in Verbal memory, so causes Autobiographical memory abnormalities	
7.	Right Anterior nucleus	Topographical and visuo-spatial Goes into closet for washroom	
8.	Bilateral medial frontal lobe involvement	Confabulations Learn different modal stimuli but cannot integrate Performance improves by cue	Usually involved in SAH (sub-arachnoid hemorrhage) due to ACOM aneurysm rupture
9.	Caudate infarct	Sudden-onset Fronto-temporal dementia • Apathy • Behavior changes • Compulsive behavior • Disinhibition • Sweet tooth	Due to interruption of caudate and frontal circuits—MPFC, OPFC, ACC

3. PPA: PRIMARY PROGRESSIVE APHASIA

	Disorder	C/F	MRI
1.	SvPPA Semantic variant of primary progressive aphasia	**Anomia** **Surface dyslexia** Initially fluent speech, but Later **word finding difficulty** The patient replaces specific names by more general words • So, they will say this "thing" instead of "glass of water" • This "fish" instead of "alligator" Same way—correctly pronounces general words • But difficulty in complex words NeuroPsychology Testing • Attention—normal • Repetition—normal • Memory—normal • Visuo-spatial—normal • ***Fluency—reduced** • ***Picture naming—reduced**	Left anterior temporal involvement (L>>R) Pathological, both AD and FTLD pathology may be seen in SvPPA Figure 11.1 MRI brain in SvPPA showing predominant temporal atrophy.
2.	LvPPA Logopenic variant	***Hesitant speech** ***Word finding difficulty** Single word comprehension normal, but Struggle with sentence comprehension And sentence **repetition*** Fluency is in b/w svPPA—and PNFA Difficulty in cappuccino, hippopotamus NeuroPsychology testing • Attention—normal • ***Repetition—impaired** • Memory—normal • Visuo-spatial—normal • Single word comprehension normal • ***Fluency—reduced** • ***Phonological paraphasia**	Posterior temporal/Inferior Parietal involvement Left posterior, Middle and superior temporal gyri and Inferior parietal regions Figure 11.2 MRI brain in LvPPA showing posterior temporal-parietal atrophy.
		Both svPPA and lvPPA will score about 75–80 on ACE-III tests, so become difficult to differentiate. Remember • Fluency is lower in logopenic variant of PPA • Single word comprehension is normal, and repetition impaired in lvPPA	

(Continued)

(Continued)

	Disorder	C/F	MRI
3.	Agrammatic PNFA Primary non-fluent aphasia	**Agrammatism + Effortful,** halting speech + Difficulty in comprehension of syntactically difficult sentences **Normal single word** comprehension Normal object knowledge	
4.	PP-AOS Primary progressive apraxia of speech	**Apraxia*** Thinks normally of words But **struggles to get it out** Slow rate of speech Distorted sounds **"Trial and error" articulation "Articulatory groping" "Segmentation"** of syllables **Yes/NO** reversal May later develop VSNG palsy	Hypo-metabolism in superior, lateral pre-motor cortex and SMA (supplementary motor area) May gradually develop PSP-CBD phenotype **Most common cause: CBD** pathology
		Mnemonic: There is **false start** and **SGT reversal** in AOS **S** = Slow speech with false starts **S** = Segmentation of speech **G** = Grouping of words (articulatory grouping) **T** = Trial and error Reversal of Yes/NO	

	Fluency	*Repetition*	*Comprehension*
Broca's aphasia	Non-fluent	Impaired	Normal
Transcortical motor aphasia		Normal	
Transcortical sensory aphasia	Fluent	Normal	Impaired
Wernicke's aphasia		Impaired	
Conduction aphasia		Impaired	Normal

Figure 11.3   Differentiating between different types of aphasia.

4. CCAS: CEREBELLAR COGNITIVE AFFECTIVE SYNDROME

Definition of CCAS	Neuro-psychological abnormalities

CCAS: Cerebellar cognitive affective syndrome: Seen in
Congenital and acquired cerebellar abnormalities
Cognitive and affective disorders in children
 	
Described by Schmahmann et al.
	• Linguistic difficulties
	• Personality changes (blunting of affect)
	• Dis-inhibition
	• Impaired spatial cognition
	• Executive dysfunction
	  • Abnormal planning, set shifting,
	  • Abstract and working memory
	
	Usually static—rarely may progress

5. ELDERLY DEGENERATIVE DEMENTIAS

		Clinical features	MRI/PET features
1.	LBD/DLBD Dementia with Lewy bodies	**The classical feature of LDB is:** **Visual hallucinations** • Helps in diagnosis of LBD • But absence of hallucinations does not rule out DLB **Visuo-spatial dysfunction*** • Absence in early stages has a 90% NPV (negative predictive value) for LBD	**Cingulate island sign**: Seen on FDG–PET, preservation of post-cingulate gyrus FDA-approved drugs • Dementia: Only RIVAstigmine • Psychosis: Pimvanserine
2.	AD Alzheimer disease	Most common dementia Involvement of bilateral temporal lobes and pre-cuneus is classical of AD Temporal lobe involvement results in a predominant amnestic syndrome Earliest involvement may be seen in Gyrus rectus In a patient <65 years: AD >> FTD/VasD Most common dementia is AD Secong common is FTD Last is vascular dementia	 Figure 11.4 MRI coronal and PET imaging in a patient with AD.
3.	PCA Posterior cortical atrophy	Variant of AD Episodic memory is preserved but patient has • Perceptual deficits • Gerstman syndrome + • Alexia, apraxia + • Visuo-spatial syndrome • Balint syndrome Insight is preserved Personality and behavior are preserved D/D: Heidenhain CJD Most common early symptom: Visuo-spatial Most common early sign: Clock drawing abnormality	 Figure 11.5 Sagittal and coronal MRI in a patient with PCA. Amyloid-tau discordance Amyloid-PET: GLOBAL deposits Tau-PET: Posterior cortical deposits

(Continued)

(Continued)

		Clinical features	MRI/PET features

4.	NPH
	Normal
	pressure
	hydrocephalus
		Earliest and Most common
		symptom: Gait apraxia
		(Bruns ataxia)
		Followed by: Memory
		impairment
		Urinary urgency enough
		for diagnosis
		Obstructive sleep apnea:
		Valsavsa @ night may
		aggravate hydrocephalus
			Ventriculomegaly Sulcal effacement
			Caudate hypometabolism**
			**DESH = tight high convexity with enlarged
			sylvian fissure
			  • Ventriculomegaly
			  • Evans index >0.3

		CSF tap test for NPH:
		  • CSF is made @ 0.3 mL/min, so replenished in 3 hours
		  • Remove 30 mL CSF—re-assess in 30 minutes	

5.	CAA	Cerebral amyloid angiopathy also sometimes presents with Convexity SAH Clinically may present with transient migratory sensory symptoms	

6. NPH: FEATURES OF DESH

  a. Ventriculomegaly.
  b. Enlarged CSF fissures: Sylvian fissure, calcarine fissure, Parieto-occipital sulcus with
    i. Secondary compression of adjacent sulci
    ii. Displacement of CSF at convexity: Hence, sulci gives tight sulci look

Good prognosis factors in NPH	Poor response to shunting in NPH
Gait apraxia onset before or same time with dementia	Dementia onset before gait apraxia
Gait abnormality is the most imp Indication for shunt	>2 years dementia
H/o head injury, meningitis, SAH	H/o alcohol abuse
DESH on MRI High convexity tightness predicts shunt response	

| FTD
Fronto-temporal
dementia | Mnemonic: A-B-C-D-E-F (50–80%)
Less common
  • Motor neuron disease (seen in
    TDP pathology)
  • Oculomotor abnormalities (if
    Midbrain involved—PSP or CBD
    pathology)
  • Semantic aphasia: Anterior
    temporal (TDP-c pathology)
  • Episodic amnesia: MTL (TDP-a or
    b pathology)
  • PNFA: Left frontal operculum
    (CBD or PSP) | 20% FTD are due to genetic
mutations

Most common—c90rf72:
Hexanucleotide repeats |

bvFTD clinical features mnemonic: (A-B-C-D-E-F) and its localization		
Apathy	Medial frontal + Anterior cingulate (ACC)	Very common (80%): Can be any pathology
Binge eating (change in eating)	Anterior insula + hypothalamus	
Compulsive behavior	Ventral striatum- pallidum	
Dis-inhibition	Orbitofrontal cortex (OPFC) + ACC	
Empathy/sympathy loss	Anterior temporal + anterior insula	Seen in 30–50%
Frontal dys-executive syndrome	Dorso-lateral prefrontal cortex (DLPFC)	

7. EARLY-ONSET AD (<65 YEARS)

a. It is the most common cause of dementia in <65 years.
b. Almost 5–6% of all AD patients present <65 years.
   (mnemonic: 5–6% < 6–5 years)
c. *Most common phenotype: Lv PPA (*repetition reduced).
d. More genetic abnormalities seen in this group.
e. More familial cases seen, most are Autosomal Dominant.
f. Usually associated with atypical features: Seizures, myoclonus, pseudobulbar palsy.
g. Hyperreflexia is seen.
h. *More mortality.
i. *More premature deaths.
j. *More common history of trauma or TBI encountered.
k. Less history of atherosclerotic/ASCVD factors.
l. But still diagnosis is late: Frequently delayed due to missed diagnosis, atypical features.
m. NeuroPsychology testing
   ● Less amnestic features
   ● Less episodic memory loss, less semantic memory loss
   ● More executive, visuo-spatial and language dysfunction
n. MRI: More widespread atrophy—involves parietal lobe also.
   ● More prominent atrophy of post-cingulate gyrus in early-onset v/s medial tempo-ral lobe in late-onset AD.

8. AD PATHOLOGY ESSENTIAL POINTS

Braak and Braak	Gave staging of AD
Senile plaques	Aggregated amyloid beta 1st deposited in neocortex Then spread sequentially
Apo-E E2/E2	Protective against AD (OR = 0.5)
Apo-E E4	Risk factor for AD—late-onset AD
Primary age-related taupathy	NFT ++ (neurofibrillary tangles) But no amyloid plaques
AgGD: Argyrophilic grain disease	Coiled bodies, tufted, balloon neurons seen on biopsy

9. AUTOIMMUNE DEMENTIAS

a) LG-I1-related encephalitis: Onset @60 years.
b) 60% have hyponatremia.
c) LGI-1: Leucine-rich glioma-inactivated antibody.
d) Most common cause of antibody mediated encephalopathy in >50 years.
e) Classical feature is: FBDS: facio-brachial dystonic seizures.

10. CHRONIC TRAUMATIC ENCEPHALOPATHY (CTE)

a. Is a taupathy.
b. 15% cases show cavum septum pellucidum (fluid-filled space).
c. Probably, due to head trauma–induced fluid waves.
d. Pathognomonic feature for diagnosis as compared to other taupathies.
   i. Accumulation of perivascular tau @ sulcal depts.
   ii. D/b CTE and DLB.
      ● Both cause dementia + parkinsonism.
      ● But CTE has dis-inhibition and explosivity.

11. HIPPOCAMPAL SCLEROSIS MAY BE SEEN IN

a. Anoxic brain injury
b. CTE
c. FTD
d. TLE (temporal lobe epilepsy)
e. OSA (obstructive sleep apnea)
f. Hippocampal sclerosis of ageing seen in **ARTERIOSCLEROSIS!**
g. Hippocampal Sclerosis + Intra-Cytoplasmic TDP-43 Inclusions in CA-1: Seen in FTD

12. TREATMENT OF DEMENTIAS

a. Conventional and atypical anti-psychotics: Have increased morbidity and mortality in all dementia.
b. Benzodiazepines: Also worsen cognition + sedating.
c. **Rx of agitation and aggression in AD**
   i. Memantine has been shown to be effective when combined with donepezil.
   ii. 1st line: SSRI and SNRI also have a +(positive) effect on mood, anxiety and agitation.
   iii. Do not use TCA—due to their anticholinergic properties.
d. **Acetylcholinesterase inhibitors**
   i. These drugs Increase secretions and decrease all pressures (Blood pressure, Intraocular pressure).
   ii. Thus, we should use with caution in patients with bradycardia.
e. **Pimvanserine.**
   i. Is a new drug.
   ii. Mechanism: 5HT-2a antagonist, no dopaminergic effect.
   iii. FDA-approved for Parkinson's disease—psychosis.
   iv. Clozapine and quetiapine used in PD-psychosis but are not FDA approved.
f. **RBD: REM sleep behavior disorder**
   i. Treatment of choice: Melatonin.
   ii. Clonazepam is used commonly, but caution in 3 groups of patients
      ● Dementia.
      ● Gait disorders.
      ● OSA.

Drug	Mechanism	Dose
Donepezil	Selective Acetylcholinesterase inhibitor	Start @ 5mg daily Goal is to reach 10 mg in 4 weeks
Galantamine	Acetylcholinesterase inhibitor Allosteric nictotine receptor modulator	Start @ 4mg twice a day Increase in 4 mg increments Goal is to reach 12 mg twice a day
Galantamine ER		Start @ 8mg daily Goals is to reach 24 mg/ day
Rivastigmine oral	Mixed Acetylcholinesterase inhibitor Butyrylcholinesterase inhibitor	Start @ 1.5 mg twice a day Increase by 1.5 mg every month Goal is to reach 6 mg twice a day
Rivastigmine patch	Transdermal patch	Start @ 4.6 mg daily Increase in 4 weeks to maximum 9.5 mg/day
Memantine	Non-competitive Glutamate NMDA antagonist	Start @ 5mg per day Can increase by 5 mg every week Maximum dose 10 mg twice a day
Memantine ER		Start @ 7 mg per day Increase every week till 28 mg/day

Figure 11.6   Drugs used in treatment of dementia.

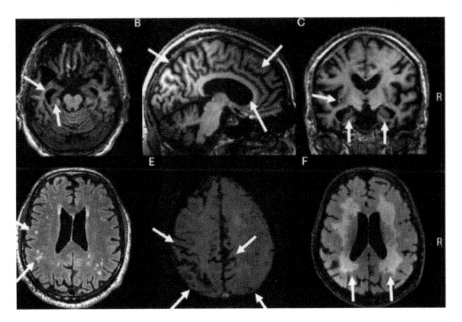

Figure 11.7   MRI findings in Alzheimer's disease (AD). Tl-weighted images demonstrate prominent hippocampal and medial temporal lobe atrophy, moderate diffuse cortical atrophy and ventricular enlargement in an 81 year old with AD dementia, subsequently confirmed at autopsy. D(FLAIR) sequence demonstrates sub-cortical and periventricular white matter hyperintensities in a 78 year old with a clinical diagnosis of AD, likely representing comorbid small vessel ischemic disease. E, Hallmarks of CAA, including scattered microbleeds and superficial siderosis, are revealed on (SWI) in a 75 year old with acute altered mental status superimposed on progressive memory and executive dysfunction. F, Confluent WM hyperintensities on FLAIR in a 75 year old with pathology-proven severe cerebral amyloid angiopathy and AD neuropathology.

NEUROSURGERY

Abbreviations

- *CSF*: Cerebrospinal fluid
- *DOC*: Drug of choice
- *LOC*: Loss of consciousness
- *ICP*: Intracranial pressure
- *MAP*: Mean arterial pressure
- *MVA*: Motor vehicle accident
- *RFA*: Radiofrequency ablation
- *SCI*: Spinal cord injury
- *SDH*: Subdural hemorrhage

1. IMPORTANT EXAM POINTS FOR NEUROSURGERY AND CRITICAL CARE

Important points asked in exams related to neurosurgical and critical care topics.

   a. HEAD INJURY followed by CSF leak.
     i. **Beta transferrin is found in CSF and inner ear** peri-lymph.
     ii. It is not found in nose, nasal secretions, ear secretions or blood.
     iii. Hence, it is a sensitive and specific marker of CSF and perilymph.
     iv. So any nasal discharge having positivity for beta transferrin is likely to be CSF.
   b. Head injury: Criteria for head CT scan (see NICE guidelines at the end of this chapter).

CT within 1 hour if	CT within 8 hours if
a. GCS <13 on initial assessment	a. Age >65 years
b. GCS <15 after 2 hours	b. Bleeding disorder
c. Suspected open skull fracture	c. Clotting disorder
d. Suspected depressed skull fracture	d. >30 minutes retrograde amnesia
e. Signs of basal skull fracture	e. Dangerous mechanism of injury
f. Post-trauma seizure	
g. Focal neurological deficits	
h. >1 episode of vomiting	
Factors increasing risk of seizure	
a. Age >65 years	
b. Early post-traumatic seizure	
c. SDH	
d. Skull fracture	
e. Contusion	
f. LOC or amnesia >24 hours	
g. Family h/o seizure	

DOI: 10.1201/b23306-12

    c. **AMANTADINE**: Some randomized trials have shown that Amantadine improves level of consciousness in trauma patients with prolonged post-traumatic unconsciousness.

    d. Cervical SCI: Significance of injury at different levels.

        i.   High cervical SCI: **C1–C4: 85%** risk of pneumonia in 1st month.

        ii. Low cervical: C5–C8 injury: 50% risk of pneumonia.

Prognosis of ambulation after SCI depends on
a. Lower ASIA score (most important factor)*
b. Neurological level of SCI (most important factor)*
c. Younger age
d. Lower extremity motor score
e. Presence of pinprick sensation (preserved sensation)—signifies incomplete SCI

    e. **Stroke and Vascular neurology**: Decompressive craniectomy indications.

        i.   Done within **24 hours**** or maximum 48 hours.

        ii. Patient has to be referred within 24 hours.

        iii. Treated within 48 hours.

        iv. Main indication is a patient with MCA stroke.

        v. Who has NIHSS >15.

        vi. And drop in GCS (with score >/=**1 in Q1a**).

        vii. CT/MRI showing >50% MCA (NCCT) involvement, >145 cm^2 on MRI-diffusion scan.

    f. Biopsy in CNS angiitis should involve

        i.   Area of abnormality on neuroimaging.

        ii. Leptomeninges.

        iii. Cerebral cortex.

    g. Brain tumours

        i.   Most common brain tumour: Metastasis/secondaries.

        ii. Most common metastasis to brain: Lung cancer in 50%.

        iii. In elderly patients, Ring-enhancing lesions, but without fever: Consider metastasis.

        iv. Brain tumours and epilepsy: Ganglioglioma: 40% of all epileptogenic tumours.

        v. Optic pathway gliomas

            a. Seen in NF-1 (neurofibromatosis 1) >> TSc (tuberous sclerosis; rare).

            b. Develops in 15–20% in children with NF-1, uncommonly may develop in adolescence.

            c. Cause visual loss and exophthalmos.

    h. Botox injections given in which muscles

Injury	Muscle botox
i. Equinovarus (Plantar flex + inverted)	Posterior tibialis + Gastro soleus
ii. Toe clawing	FHL and FDL

2. COMPLICATIONS IN NEURO-CRITICAL CARE

CIM and CIP in ICU

CIM = Critical illness myopathy
CIP = Critical illness polyneuropathy

    a. Occurs in presence of sepsis or SIRS or septic encephalopathy.

    b. Prevalence of CIM is more common than >>> CIP.

    c. CIP is sensory + motor axonal (distal) polyneuropathy.

d. Risk factors for CIM/CIP
    i. Prolonged ICU stay.
    ii. Sepsis, SIRS, multi-organ failure.
    iii. Drugs: Steroid use and non-depolarizing muscle-blocking agents.
e. Clinically, patients have distal muscle weakness + atrophy + wasting.
f. There may be delayed weaning off the ventilator.
g. Sometimes CIP and CIM can occur together.
h. Then it is difficult to differentiate both.

Lance–Adams Syndrome: Post-Hypoxic Myoclonus

a. Occurs in case of hypoxic brain injury.
b. Complication of a successful cardio-pulmonary resuscitation.
c. Patients have mainly action myoclonus.
d. Rx.

Will help in hypoxic myoclonus	NOT helpful
a. Valproate	a. Amantadine
b. Levetiracetam	b. Phenytoin
c. Piracetam	c. Nitrazepam
d. Clonazepam	d. Phenobarbitone
	e. Primidone
	f. Amitriptyline/NorTriptyline/Vasopressin

Brain Death

a. For assessing **brain death, ensure of the following parameters:**
    a. Core temp >34° C
    b. MAP >60 mmHg
    c. pH 7.35–7.45
    d. $paCO_2$ <6 Kpa
    e. paO_2 >10 Kpa
    f. Serum sodium: 115–160 mEq/L
    g. Serum potassium >2 mEq/L
    h. Phosphate levels 0.5–3 mEq/L
    i. Magnesium levels 0.5–3 mEq/L
    j. Blood glucose 3–20 mmol/L

3. COMMON NEUROLOGICAL SCALES USED IN ICU

EGRIS: Erasmus GBS Respiratory Insufficiency Score

a. Predicts respiratory insufficiency in GBS.
b. 3 criteria used
    i. Days between onset of weakness and hospitalization.
    ii. Facial weakness or bulbar weakness.
    iii. MMRC weakness grade—sum score.
c. Low risk if score is 0–2.
d. Intermediate risk if score is 3–4.
e. High risk if score is 5–7.

FOUR Score

a. Full Outline of UnResponsiveness score
(see Table 12.2 for calculation of FOUR score)
b. Higher inter-rater reliability than GCS (Glasgow Coma Scale)

Table 12.1 EGRIS Score

Days between onset of weakness and hospital admission	>7 days	0
	4–7 days	1
	<3 days	2
Facial and/or bulbar weakness at the time of admission	Absent	0
	Present	1
MRC sum score at the time of admission	60–51	0
	50–41	1
	40–31	2
	30–21	3
	<21	4
Total score		0–7

Table 12.2 FOUR Score

Components	Findings	Score
Eye response	Eyelids open, tracking or blinking to commands	4
	Eyelids open but not tracking	3
	Eyelids closed, but open to loud noise	2
	Eyelids closed, but open to pain	1
	Eyelids remain closed despite pain	0
Motor response	Makes sign (thumbs up, fist, peace sign)	4
	Localizing to pain	3
	Flexion in response to pain	2
	Extension in response to pain	1
	No response to pain or generalized myoclonic status	0
Brainstem reflexes	Pupils and corneal reflex present	4
	One pupil is dilated (wide and fixed)	3
	Pupils or corneal reflex absent	2
	Pupils and corneal reflex absent	1
	Pupils and corneal and cough reflex are all absent	0
Respiration	Not intubated, regular breathing pattern	4
	Not intubated, Cheyne–Stokes breathing pattern	3
	Not intubated, irregular breathing pattern	2
	Breathes above ventilator rate	1
	Breathes at ventilator rate or apnea	0

ICAT

   a. Intensive care after thrombolysis score.

   b. Predicting ICU requirement after IV thrombolysis in an acute stroke patient

      i. ICAT >/= 2 increases ICU requirement by 13 times.

      ii. ICAT >5 predicts ICU requirement by 94% specificity.

      iii. Easy way to remember: Black male with high BP and high NIHSS requires ICU more.

Table 12.3 ICAT Score

Components		Score
Sex	Female	0
	Male	1
Black race	No	0
	Yes	1
Systolic blood pressure	<160 mmHg	0
	160–200 mmHg	1
	>200 mmHg	2
NIHSS	<6	0
	7–12	1
	>13	2
Total score		0–8

4. COMMON EEG FINDINGS IN ICU

a. Alpha coma
   i. Seen in unresponsive or comatose patients or Hypoxic ischemic encephalopathy.
   ii. The EEG background is similar to alpha frequency, but there is no reactivity as seen in normal alpha.
   iii. Complete form + Lack of reactivity to noxious stimuli.
   iv. Indicates Poor prognosis.

b. Burst suppression
   i. Periods of high-voltage EEG (called bursts).
   ii. Interspersed with periods of no activity (suppression).
   iii. Found in
      • HIE.
      • Hypothermia.
      • Anesthetic coma.

c. **Poor prognostic findings in EEG**
   i. Alpha coma.
   ii. Burst suppression pattern.
   iii. Voltage suppression <10 mcV >24 h.
   iv. Myoclonic Status epilepticus.

5. COMMON RADIOLOGY FINDINGS IN ICU

a. **Hypoglycemic encephalopathy**
   i. Risk factors: Diabetic patients on Insulin therapy, Alcoholic patients.
   ii. MRI shows: T2 hyperintensity in cortex and basal ganglia.
   iii. Corresponding diffusion restriction is seen in these areas.
   iv. **Parieto-occipital cortex and insula involvement**** is classical for hypoglycemia.

b. **Hyper-ammonemic** or porto-systemic encephalopathy
   i. Some findings are similar to hypoglycemia.
   ii. But there is more prominent involvement of frontal cortex.
   iii. **More globus pallidi**** **involvement.**

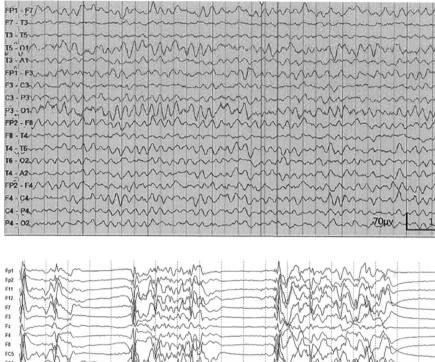

Figures 12.1 and 12.2   EEGs showing alpha coma and burst suppression.

c. **Hypoxic** encephalopathy
   i. Diffuse cortical and deep Gray matter involvement.
   ii. **Peri-Rolandic cortex (Most common site)** + thalami involvement is classical.
   iii. Isolated Basal ganglia involvement may be seen.
   iv. Watershed zone involvement.
   v. Cerebellum.
   vi. Gray matter has higher oxygen and metabolic requirement.
   vii. Oxygen and glucose needed to supply large number of synapses in gray matter. Hence, these are the areas to be involved preferentially in hypoxic insult.

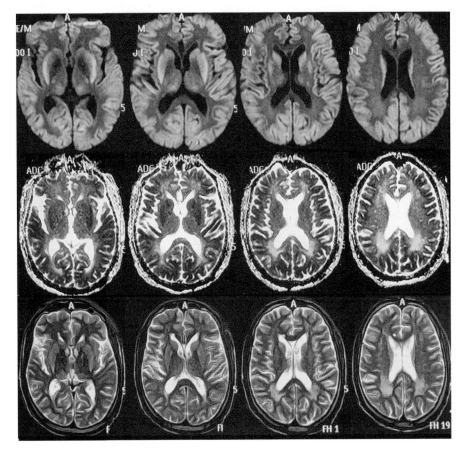

Figure 12.3 MRI brain diffusion (top panel), ADC (middle panel) and T2 (lower panel) images showing evidence of hypoxic ischemic encephalopathy.

Signs of Hypoxia Described in Neuroradiology

a. **Reversal sign on non-contrast CT**: Reversal of normal CT attenuation of Gray and white matter.

b. **White cerebellum sign**: Diffuse edema and hypoattenuation of cortex; sparing brainstem and cerebellum. Hence cerebellum appears more hyperdense than cortex.

c. **Cortical laminar necrosis**: Linear hyperdensity outlining the cortex and cortical enhancement.

d. **Pseudo-SAH**: Due to cerebral edema and reduced attenuation of cortex, but engorgement of veins due to high ICP—then sub-arachnoid space appears white—appearing as sub-arachnoid bleed.

6. NICE GUIDELINES: SCIATIA OR LOW BACKACHE

a. Sciatica without red flags: Discharge with analgesics.
   i. EPIDURAL INJECTION: In acute cases.
   ii. RFA: In chronic cases.
   iii. Spinal injection and spinal fusion: Not recommended.
   iv. Spinal decompression: In refractory cases.

Main topic	Explanation in NICE guidelines	
Risk assessment	The risk assessment tool used for sciata is:	STarT Back
	SBST: Keel's STarT Back Screening Tool: • 9-item version • Brief and validated screening tool for sciatica	
Imaging for sciatica	Do not offer imaging in non-specialist set-up Explain to the patient that they may not need imaging even after referral	
	When to do imaging • Imaging done only in specialist set-up (MSK clinic or hospital) • Done only if it will change the management	
Rx: Self-management	Provide advice and information tailored to needs of patient Encourage to continue with ADL (activities of daily living)	
Exercises	Group exercise programme (biomechanical, aerobic, mind–body or a combination of approaches) within the NHS	
Orthotics	**DO NOT OFFER** • Corsets or belts • Foot orthotics • Rocker sole shoes • Traction for Low backache	
Physiotherapy	Consider manual therapy (spinal manipulation, mobilization or soft tissue techniques such as massage)—but only with exercise treatment	
Others	**DO NOT offer** • Acupuncture • USG (ultrasound therapy) • PENS • TENS • Interferential therapy	
Cognitive Behavior Therapy/Psychotherapy	**Offered only along with exercise +/– manual therapy**	
Combined therapy	**Consider combined (manual + psychotherapy) when** • Failed previous treatment • Significant psycho-social obstructions	
Medication of sciatica	**DO NOT offer** • **Gabapentin/Pregabalin** • **Benzodiazepines** • **Antiepileptic therapy** • **Steroids** • **TCA, SSRI, SNRI (antidepressants)** • **Opioids for acute/chronic low backache/ sciatica**	No benefit of these medicines
If already taking these medicines	Explain the risk of continuing listed medications Consider tapering and stopping these medicines	
NSAIDs**	Explain limited benefit and/or harm of NSAIDs Take into account the gastric, liver and cardio renal toxicity with respect to age of patient Use lowest dose possible For least time	DO NOT give Paracetamol alone

Main topic	Explanation in NICE guidelines	
Opioids	Weak opioids +/– Paracetamol if NSAIDs contraindicated	
Non-surgical management	Spinal injection: DO not offer spinal injection for low backache	
Radiofrequency denervation	For Chronic Low backache • If Other treatments have not worked • Moderate to severe pain (Visual analogue score >5) • Main source of pain is structures supplied by **medial branch** nerve	
	Neuroimaging not a pre-requisite for planning patient for RF Do a diagnostic medial branch block Offer RFD only if a positive response to diagnostic block	
Epidural injection	Can be used for acute severe sciatica Epidural injection along with steroids DO NOT offer for central canal stenosis/neurogenic claudication	
Surgical decompression	Considered If non-surgical treatment has not helped Imaging suggestive of sciatica symptoms Do not allow age, BMI, smoking status to influence surgery	
Spinal fusion	DO NOT offer these treatment options	
Disk replacement		

7. NICE GUIDELINES: SPINAL CORD INJURY (SCI)

Initial assessment	<C> ABCDE • Cervical spine • Airway • Breathing • Circulation	<C>ABCDE Can have both these full forms
	Catastrophic hemorrhage Airway with in-line spinal immobilization Breathing Circulation Disability (neurological) Exposure and environment	
At all stages	Protect Cervical spine with manual in-line spinal immobilization Avoid moving remainder of spine	
Full in-line immobilization if	Under influence of alcohol, drugs Confused or uncooperative patient Low GCS Spinal pain Hand or foot weakness Altered absent sensation Priapism H/o past spinal problems	

Spine assessment		
Assess C-spine	Using Canadian C-spine rule	
High risk of C-spine injury	**Low risk of C-spine injury**	**No risk**
>65 years	If they have 1 of	If they have one of the low risk factor but
Paresthesia in UL/LL	• Minor rear end MVA	Able to actively rotate neck 45 degrees
Dangerous mechanism • Fall from >1 meter height • Fall from >5 steps • Head-on collision • Diving • Horse riding • High-speed motor MVA • Ejection from motor vehicle • Rollover motor vehicle • Accident involving recreational motor vehicle	• Comfortable in sitting • Ambulatory • Delayed-onset neck pain • No midline Cervical tenderness • Unable to actively rotate neck to 45 degrees	
Canadian C-spine rule is difficult to apply in children		

Assess thoracic or Lumbar Spine injury
Assessment particularly important in: 1. >65 years age 2. Pre-existing spinal abnormality 3. Risk of osteoporosis—example steroid users 4. Suspected spinal fracture at another level
5. Dangerous mechanism of injury • Fall >3 meters • Load on buttocks • Lap belt restraint only • Horse riding • High-speed MVA/Ejection • Recreational motorized vehicle
6. Abnormal neurological signs and symptoms
7. Abnormal neurological exam • Motor or sensory signs • Deformity or midline tenderness • Bony midline tenderness on percussion • Midline or spinal pain on cough
8. On mobilization—patient experiences pain—sit stand step walk—stop if pain
Full in-line spinal immobilization
Carry out full in-line spinal immobilization if • High-risk C-spine injury • Low-risk C-spine injury + not able to rotate 45 degrees • Risk of thoracic or Lumbo-Sacral injury
Spinal immobilization is difficult in • Short neck, wide neck patients • Pre-existing spinal deformity • Uncooperative people, children, agitated patients
Spinal immobilization can be counter-productive if • It Increases pain • Worsen Focal neuro-deficits

How to do
• Fit appropriately **sized semi-rigid collar** (unless any contraindications like: Compromised airway, spinal deformity as in ankylosing spondylitis) • Re-assess airway after applying • Place and secure person on scoop stretcher • Secure person with head tape and block—ideally vacuum mattress
In children
• Consider involving family members • Keep infants in their car seats
Extrication
• Ask to self-extricate if possible • Use long board only for extrication, not transport

Further Management of Pain	Assess with any scale suitable for pain **IV morphine** is the DOC** Ketamine is the 2nd DOC If no IV access—**nasal atomized diamorphine** or ketamine	DOC = drug of choice
Transport	Directly to a major trauma center Not necessary to transport to Spinal cord injury center If emergency—Rapid sequence/intubation needed • Shift to the nearest trauma center	
Imaging	For suspected SCI—imaging is done on emergency basis Should be analyzed by a health care worker	
Children	<16 years—MRI spine is done if high-risk SCI (by Canadian C-spine rule) Based on motor or sensory deficits If none of these—plain X-ray is sufficient If head injury—follow head injury guidelines	
Adults >16	Do CT spine If CT normal but neuro deficit are present—then do MRI spine	
Thoraco-lumbar-sacral spine injury	1st line—do X-ray spine If abnormal—do CT spine If any fracture suspected—image rest of Spinal cord	
Polytrauma	Do whole body scannogram + CT	
Communication	With specialist neurosurgeon or spinal surgeon In case of SCI: Communication has to be done	**Within 4 hours**

Medication	DO NOT use
	  • Steroids
	  • Nimodipine
	  • Naloxone
	  • Neuropathic drugs	

Summary	A summary about the patient with action plan Sent to GP	**Within 24 hours**

8. NICE GUIDELINES: TRAUMATIC BRAIN INJURY (TBI)

Initial assessment	GCS—Glasgow Coma Scale	
For children	We use pediatric Glasgow Coma Scale (GCS) In pediatric GCS—we use grimace instead of verbal response	
If GCS <8	Inform the emergency department while on the way Inform the anesthetist so that critical care team gets involved in airway management	
ER management	Patient should be immediately assessed by trained staff For patients in ER who have GCS <15 Have to be immediately assessed by a trained member of staff For GCS <8 Ensure early involvement of an appropriately trained clinician to provide advanced airway management	Within 15 min
	If C-spine injury or TBI suspected—extend to full assessment To see the need of imaging If no major injury suspected: To be evaluated by clinician	Within 1 hour
Pain management	Manage properly to avoid increase in ICP • Immobilization • Splintage • Low-dose opioids	
Involve neurosurgeon in management if	• GCS <8 • Confusion >4 hours • Worsening of GCS after admission • FND (focal neuro deficits) • Seizures without full recovery • Penetrating injury • CSF leak Also, neurosurgeon should be called when the imaging shows "significant surgical abnormalities" The definition of these abnormalities has to be developed by local hospital	
CT scan	Initial investigation of choice Try to minimize radiation If CT facility is not available, arrange transfer to another suitable hospital	

CT within 1 hour done if	CT within 8 hours done if
a. GCS <13 on initial assessment b. GCS <15 after 2 hours c. Suspected open skull fracture d. Suspected depressed skull fracture e. Signs of basal skull fracture f. Post-trauma seizures g. FND h. >1 episode of vomiting	1. >65 years 2. Bleeding disorder 3. Clotting disorder 4. Anticoagulants 5. Warfarin/acitrom/NOACs 6. >30 minutes retrograde amnesia 7. Dangerous mechanism of injury

Radiology report should be available in **one hour**

Initial assessment	GCS—Glasgow Coma Scale	

CT within 1 hour (child)	CT within 1 hour of >1 of
a. **GCS <14 on initial assessment** b. **GCS <15 for infants** c. GCS <15 after 2 hours d. Suspected open skull fracture e. Suspected depressed skull fracture f. Signs of basal skull fracture g. Post-trauma seizure h. FND i. **Swelling or laceration >5 cm on head**	1. LOC >5 min 2. Abnormal drowsiness 3. >3 e/o vomiting 4. Amnesia >5 min 5. Dangerous injury

Radiology report should be available in **one hour**	
MRI brain	MRI brain is not the preferred imaging in a patient with TBI
X-ray skull	Do not use X-ray skull in patients aged >16 years

C-spine—What Investigation to do?	
CT spine	When area of concern or uncertainty on X-ray Review occipital condyles Review the scan in bone window
MRI spine	MRI is done when neurological examination shows signs and symptoms—suspecting of C-spine injury
MR/CT Angiography	Suspicion of vascular injury • Vertebral malalignment, • Fracture involving the foramina transversaria or lateral processes, • Posterior circulation syndrome
Foramen magnum scans to be done	If lower cranial nerve palsies are seen in dangerous accident

CT spine within 1 hour if	
• GCS <13 • Intubated patient • Plain X-ray technically in adequate • Plain X-ray suspicious • Polytrauma • Imaging of cervical spine is needed before surgery • Or high-risk C-spine (see Canadian C-spine rule)	
None of these	Urgent X-ray in 3 planes within 1 hour

Refer	
To neurosurgical care if	GCS <8
Intubate all patients whose	GCS <8
Also intubate if	Coma Loss of protective laryngeal reflex Irregular respiration Hypoxia paO$_2$ <13 Hypercarbia paCO$_2$ >6 Hyperventilation causing paCO$_2$ <4
Intubate during transfer if	Deteriorating GCS (1 point or more on motor scale) Unstable facial fracture Copious bleeding from mouth—base of skull fracture Seizures

(Continued)

(Continued)

C-spine—What Investigation to do?	
Goals during transfer	Intubate using muscle relaxant and short acting sedation Appropriate analgesia and muscle relaxant to be given The hemodynamic aims/goals are: • MAP >80 mmHg • paO_2 >13 kPa • $paCO_2$ 4.5–5 kPa
Before transfer	Transfer may be often urgent, but complete the initial resuscitation and stabilization of the person Establish comprehensive monitoring before transfer to avoid complications during the journey Do not transport someone with: • Persistent hypotension, despite resuscitation • Until the cause has been identified and they are stabilized

Transport of patient: Remote advice services (for example, NHS 111) should refer people who have sustained a head injury	
To the emergency ambulance services (that is, 999) for emergency transport to the emergency department if: • Unconscious or lack of full consciousness • Any FND • Seizures • High energy head injury	To a hospital emergency department if there are any of these risk factors: • Patient has recovered to full consciousness • Has post-injury amnesia • Persistent headache • Vomiting • H/o previous brain surgery • H/o bleeding or clotting disorder • Current drug or alcohol consumption

Admit	
If	GCS <15 Imaging shows any abnormality CT needed but not possible urgently Severe headache, vomiting Seizures Intoxication CSF leak, shock Ongoing post-traumatic amnesia Meningismus Suspected non-accidental injury
Observation: Always keep a close eye on	GCS Limb movements RR (respiratory rate), HR (heart rate) • O_2 (oxygen saturation), temperature Pupil size and reaction
Observation of admitted patients	Any patient with GCS 15: Observe • ½ hourly x 2 hours • 1 hourly for 4 hours • 2 hourly after that Any patient with GCS <15: ½ hourly observation till GCS reaches 15
In the hospital	
Role of tranexamic acid	Head injury patients with GCS of 12 or less but no active extracranial bleeding: • Tranexamic acid 2 g IV bolus (adults) 15–30 mg/kg IV bolus (children <16 years)

Hypo-pituitarism	If patient has persistent hyponatremia or low blood pressure Evaluation for hypo-pituitarism may be done
Discharge	
Detailed summary includes	• Nature and severity of injury • Risk factors and need to return to ER • Details about recovery process • Contact details of community and hospital services • Details about return to activities of daily living

PAIN AND HEADACHE

Abbreviations

- *SAH*: Sub-arachnoid hemorrhage
- *CVT*: Cerebral venous thrombosis
- *RCVS*: Reversible vasoconstriction syndrome
- *CAA*: Cerebral amyloid angiopathy
- *DSA*: Digital subtraction angiography
- *GCS*: Glasgow Coma Scale
- *TMJ*: Temporo-mandibular joint

1. HEADACHE

	Disease	Causes and clinical features	Diagnosis and Rx
1.	Thunderclap headache	Defined as headache with onset and peak within 1 minute; Lasts >5 minutes Causes • SAH • CVT • RCVS • Pituitary apoplexy	Emergency NCCT (Non-contrast CT scan of head) should be done in all patients of thunderclap headache—to exclude SAH LP: Lumbar puncture (*see next row)
		If initial NCCT scan is normal: Perform **a LP after 6–12 hours**. At least 6, ideally 12 hours later • Most sensitive marker of SAH = Xanthochromia (bilirubin in CSF) • Xanthochromia is also seen in case of high CSF protein, jaundice and carotene • RBC usually decrease from 1st to 3rd sample in traumatic tap • But remain constant in case of SAH LP contraindicated if platelets: **<50,000** (American blood bank); **40,000** (British hematology)	
2.	Cortical SAH (sulcal SAH)	Causes of sulcal SAH • CVT • RCVS • CAA	

(Continued)

(Continued)

	Disease	Causes and clinical features	Diagnosis and Rx
3.	RCVS Reversible cerebral vasoconstriction syndrome	Recurrent thunderclap headaches Superficial cortical SAH Initial DSA: Angiogram may miss the diagnosis Causes • Herbal meds • Diet pill • Illicit drugs • Sertaline	**RCVS2 score: –2 to 10** (see Figure 13.1) Used to differentiate RCVS and other arteriopathies >5 high **Specificity (99%)** and **Sensitivity (90%)** for diagnosing RCVS <2 rules out RCVS

History/ examination		Points
Recurrent Thunderclap headache (single or recurrent)	Present	5
	Absent	0
Carotid involvement (Intracranial)	Affected	-2
	Not affected	0
Vasoconstriction trigger (eg drugs)	Present	3
	Absent	0
Sex	Female	1
	Male	0
Sub-arachnoid hemorrhage	Present	1
	Absent	0
Total score: <2 is negative for RCVS 3-4 is equivocal, >5 is positive for RCVS		

Figure 13.1 RCVS2 score for differentiating RCVS from other arteriopathies.

4.	Ciliary **ganglio-plegic** migraine	Headache associated with • Transient or prolonged dilated pupil • Mydriasis outlasts headache • Mean duration—3 months • Also seen in Adie pupil	Dilatation is due to cholinergic super-sensitivity Pupil reacts to 0.125% pilocarpine
5.	SMART Stroke-like migraine attacks after cranial Radiotherapy	Recurrent + prolonged hemispheric symptoms (like hemiparesis) along with Headache or seizures Symptoms usually recover Occasional permanent sequalae may be due to cortical laminar necrosis	Initial neuroimaging may be normal but MRI changes may occur in delayed Phase: 2–7 days later Gadolinium enhancement + swelling is seen in sulci and cortex of one side (unilateral)
		Clues in question will be • **History of malignancy/radiotherapy** • **Unilateral symptoms** • **Unilateral imaging findings late in course (initial MRI normal)**	

	Disease	Causes and clinical features	Diagnosis and Rx
6.	Pituitary apoplexy	Due to infarction or hemorrhage in pituitary Presents with • Thunderclap headache • Visual disturbance • Low GCS • Multiple cranial nerve palsies • Bilateral ophthalmoplegia • Low Blood pressure	Blood tests: ACTH deficiency produces dys-electrolytemia Hypo-cortisolemia So, Rx is to give urgent steroids
	FHM: Familial hemiplegic migraine: Migraine associated with transient hemiparesis/ hemiplegia along with family history of similar complaints. There are 3 types:		
7.	FHM-1	Due to gene defect in: CACNA1a Calcium channels	MRI: Cerebellar atrophy, ataxia
8.	FHM-2	ATP1a2	
9.	FHM-3	SCN1a Sodium channels	
10.	Sporadic Hemiplegic migraine	Headache associated with transient hemiparesis/hemiplegia but No family h/o migraine	
11.	Menstrual migraine	Menstruation and its related hormones can trigger headaches and migraines in women Migraine is more common in women than men	Prophylactic therapy: Start 2 days prior to menses and continue for 7 days Frovatriptan >> naratriptan or zolmitriptan For immediate relief (within 2 hours): Rizatriptan and sumatriptan
12.	Red ear syndrome	Clinically presents with • U/L ear burning pain and redness • Daily (multiple) attacks • Each attack is <1 hour • Rarely may be bilateral also Triggers: Neck movements, heat, cold, activity	Causes • Idiopathic • 55% cases are associated with migraine • Rest associated with TMJ dysfunction and Cervical spine disease No specific prophylactic Rx required
13.	MOH Medication overuse headache	Develops during the treatment of primary headache disorders Worsening headache while taking medicines for **>3 months** **Considered a secondary headache disorder**	**Criteria for diagnosis: Medicines should be taken for >10 days a month** **>10 days/month: COTE** • Combination drugs • Opioids • Triptans • Ergots **>15 days/month in case of:** NSAIDs

2. PRIMARY HEADACHE DISORDERS

	Headache	Clinical features	Investigation and Rx
	TAC	Trigeminal autonomic cephalalgias TACs start with Superior salivatory nucleus: So affect parasympathetic dilatory pathway	
1a.	SUNCT/SUNA Short-lasting unilateral neuralgiform headache with conjunctival injection and tearing	Criteria for diagnosis a. >20 episodes per day fulfilling later criteria b. Each 1–600 seconds c. Moderate to severe unilateral pain • Single stabs • Series of stabs/sawtooth • Orbital/temporal/trigeminal distribution d. 1/5 cranial autonomic symptoms • Conjunct injection or lacrimation • Nasal congestion or rhinorrhea • Eyelid edema • Forehead and facial swelling • Miosis/ptosis	Occurs at least once a day SUNCT = SUNA + Conjunctival Injection Rx: LTG (Lamotrigine) SUNA: Always assess for vascular loop compression and for pituitary abnormalities. Can get MRI brain
1b.	HC/PH Hemicrania continua or paroxysmal hemicrania	Very severe unilateral pain, (V1>V2, V3) Lasting for 1–600 seconds Causes: 23% are post-**head trauma** May also be associated with • Sinus surgery • Brain surgery • Pituitary infarct • Vitreous hemorrhage	Trigeminal neuralgia is more in V2 and V3 distribution HC/PH is more common in V1
1c.	CH Cluster headaches	Severe Unilateral orbital or temporal pain • Lasting 15–180 minutes + • 1 of the following • Conjunct injection or lacrimation • Nasal congestion or rhinorrhea • Eyelid edema • Forehead and facial swelling • Miosis/ptosis	Frequency 0.5–8 times a day Mainly pain during Night time Risk factors: Male, higher BMI Rx: Verapamil CH prophylaxis given for 2 weeks after complete cessation of symptoms: Then stop; slow taper No long-term treatment till next attack
		Surgical treatments • Peripheral sphenopalatine ganglion blockade may be efficacious in cluster headache, although evidence is not yet sufficient for this treatment • Deep brain stimulation has been tried experimentally for the treatment of cluster headache, but sufficient evidence is lacking, especially given the risks of this treatment Posterior fossa decompression and vagus nerve stimulator implantation do not have any role	

	Headache	Clinical features	Investigation and Rx
2.	CH and PH overlap	CH: 15–180 min; >8 attacks PH: 2–30 minutes; >5 attacks	So overlapping symptoms: Give **indomethacin trial first** Treatment response is the best way to differentiate between both
3.	CM Chronic migraine	Migraine x 3 months Headache for 15/more days a month Migraine features on 8/more days a month	Prophylactic therapy • Topiramate • Amitriptyline • Propranolol BotoxA: If already tried 3 different prophylactic drugs
Important aspects of migraine treatment		**Drugs and specific considerations** • Weight loss: Occurs with Topiramate • Pregnancy: Topiramate is avoided • Weight gain: Amitriptyline, pizotifen, Flunarizine • Candesartan maybe used for prophylaxis • Galcanezumab: Recommended if migraine days >**4/months**	
BotoxA response		Stop BotoxA after 2 cycles if • Not responding to BotoxA (**30% decrease** in headache days per month) • CM changed to Episodic (<15 headache days/month x 3 consecutive months)	

3. SECONDARY AND OTHER HEADACHE DISORDERS

	Headache	Clinical features	Investigation and Rx
1.	Epicrania fugax	Headache starts posteriorly Moves forward in a **straight/ zigzag line** Reaches forehead, eye or nose 1/3 will have nasal/ocular autonomic symptoms	Attacks last: 1–10 seconds Described as Electric or "stabbing" Rx: LTG (Lamotrigine) and GBP (gabapentin)
2.	Glossopharyngeal neuralgia	Starts with severe throat pain That radiates to ear or back of tongue Attack lasts few seconds Triggered by coughing or swallowing Weight loss may be an associated feature Due to connections with Vagus, it can cause • Asystole • Hypotension • Bradycardia • Palatal myoclonus	Rx • CBZ/ox-CBZ • GBP (gabapentin) • LTG (Lamotrigine) • Phenytoin Surgical: MVD (microvascular decompression) of the IX and X nerves

(Continued)

(Continued)

	Headache	Clinical features	Investigation and Rx
3.	GCA/temporal arteritis Giant cell arteritis	GCA is a disease of elderly GCA in <50 years: Is exceptionally rare So, diagnosed in patients >50 years Patients complain of headache or orbital pain or ear pain Generally, the pain is more around the eyes or near the temples 15% may have PUO	ESR is usually >50 mm/hour ESR may be <40 in some CRP may be normal Temporal artery Doppler and/or biopsy may be done Rx: Steroids urgently given to prevent vision loss
4.	Fibromyalgia	Chronic widespread pains >3 months Tender points present Criteria • WPI >/= 7 + SSS >/= 5 • WPI 4–6 + SSS >/= 9 • Symptoms >3 months • Pain in 4 of 5 regions including: Neck, back, elbow, hips, knees • **Jaw, chest and abdomen not** included • Fibromyalgia is exclusive of other diagnoses WPI = widespread pain index SSS = symptom severity scale	Fibromyalgia may co-exist with • Sleep disorders • Anxiety • PTSD • IBD (inflammatory bowel disease) • Depression • OCD Rx: Includes diet and lifestyle changes, antidepressants, behaviour therapy
5.	Primary exercise headache	Headache associated with exercise, especially Strenuous exercise in hot/high altitude Patient complains of headache, which is pulsating, frontal headache Starts <1 hour after exercise, lasts <1 hour 70% cases associated with venous congestion: IJV incompetence	Indomethacin responsive headache Indomethacin is taken 30 min before starting exercise Prolonged warm up period advised Usually, self-limiting in months to year
6.	SIH Spontaneous intracranial hypotension	Sudden onset Orthostatic headache Increased headache with upright posture Predisposing factors: Trivial trauma/ like headache started after patient recently started playing rugby	MRI: Diffuse pachymeningeal enhancement Bilateral SDH (subdural hematoma) Engorgement of venous structures Pituitary hyperemia Sagging of brain CT myelography or CE-MRI spine may be more sensitive Rx: Autologous blood patch

	Headache	Clinical features	Investigation and Rx
7.	CRPS 1,2 Complex regional pain syndrome	Clinically presents with unexplained limb pains or paresthesia associated with trophic and autonomic features: Pain is out of proportion of injury Seen Post-trauma **Allodynia** (**classical) More heat than cold Persistent deep pain which increases with movement Trophic changes of skin and nails seen Increased or decreased sweating Physical and morphological changes in limb Deformities	Orlando and Budapest criteria used for diagnosis Nerve conduction studies Type 1 CRPS: No nerve damage Type 2 CRPS: Nerve damage + Can do a nerve conduction study to look for nerve damage Rx: Counselling, antidepressants and neuropathic drugs

All of the following criteria must be met:
- Continuing pain, disproportionate to the inciting event
- 1 sign in 2 or more categories mentioned below
- 1 symptom in 3 or more categories mentioned below
- No other diagnosis can better explain the signs and symptoms

Category	Signs/ symptoms
Sensory	Allodynia and/ or hyperalgesia
Vasomotor	Temperature asymmetry and/or Skin colour changes and/or skin colour asymmetry
Sudomotor/ edema	Edema and/or sweating changes and/or sweating asymmetry
Motor/ trophic changes	Decreased range of motion and/or motor dysfunction (weakness/ tremors/ dystonia) and/or trophic changes (hair/skin/nails)

Figure 13.2   Diagnostic criteria for CRPS.

	Headache	Clinical features	Investigation and Rx

8.	LCS/LSS
	Lumbar canal stenosis or lumbar spinal stenosis
		Acquired lumbar canal stenosis due to
		• Facet hypertrophy
		Presents with
		• Back pain
		• + Radiating pain—sciatica
		• + Neurogenic claudication
		• Pain aggravated by standing and spine extension
		• Relieved by
		  • Trunk flexion
		  • Stooping
		  • Sitting or lying
			Usually presents in the elderly
			7th decade—symptomatic
			In Severe cases: Neurogenic bladder may be seen
			
			Rx: Neuropathic pain drugs
			Surgery uncommonly required
			Physiotherapy

(Continued)

(Continued)

9.	Relapsing poly-chondritis	Autoimmune systemic disease Recurrent inflammatory episodes of cartilaginous tissues Inflammation with exacerbations • Polyarthritis • + Auricular symptoms • + Eye symptoms • +/– CNS symptoms **Bilateral auricular involvement—** cartilaginous part—90% involved, but **SPARES the EAR LOBE** Eye: Scleritis, epi-scleritis, conjunctivitis seen CNS: Headache, meningitis, psychosis or CNS vasculitis Signs of meningeal irritation: Nuchal rigidity, vomiting	CSF analysis: Pleocytosis (lymphocytic or polymorphs) Rx: Autoimmune disease—so— steroids and Long-term sparing agents
10.	Occipital condyle syndrome	Severe occipital pain + Ipsilateral hypoglossal palsy Pain radiates to ipsilateral mastoid Symptoms are exaggerated by turning/tilting head to contra-lateral side Allodynia ++	Always evaluate for Skull base metastasis from • Breast cancer • Prostate cancer
11.	IgG4 disease	Autoimmune systemic disorder May present with • Hypertrophic pachymeningitis • Sarcoidosis • En-plaque meningioma • Dural thickenings • AIP: Autoimmune pancreatitis • Sclerosing cholangitis	Biopsy shows: (Hallmark features) • Lympho-plasma infiltrate • **Storiform pattern**** • **Cart-wheel**** arrangement of fibroblasts and inflammatory cells • Eosinophilia • Obliterative phlebitis

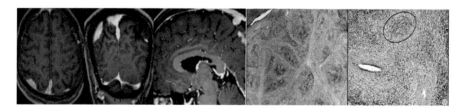

Figure 13.3   IgG4 disease: MRI brain showing pachymeningeal enhancement and biopsy showing storiform pattern.

Diagnostic criteria cut-offs		
TTH	Episodic TTH: <15 days/month	Chronic TTH: >15 days/month x 3 months
Migraine	–same–	–same–
CH	0.5–8 times a day, pain free >1 month	**Pain free <1 month** in 12-month period
Menstrual	Headache between –2 to +3 days after onset + **In at least 2 out of 3 consecutive cycles**	

Headache feature	Tension-type headache	Migraine (with or without aura)	Cluster headache
Pain location (can be in the head, face or neck)	Bilateral	Unilateral or bilateral	Unilateral (around the eye, above the eye and along the side of the head/face)
Pain quality	Pressing/tightening (non-pulsating)	Pulsating (throbbing or banging in young people aged 12 to 17 years)	Variable (can be sharp, boring, burning, throbbing or tightening)
Pain intensity	Mild or moderate	Moderate or severe	Severe or very severe
Effect on activities	Not aggravated by routine activities of daily living	Aggravated by, or causes avoidance of, routine activities of daily living	Restlessness or agitation
Other symptoms	None	Unusual sensitivity to light and/or sound or nausea and/or vomiting Symptoms of aura can occur with or without headache and: • are fully reversible • develop over at least 5 minutes • last 5 to 60 minutes Typical aura symptoms include visual symptoms such as flickering lights, spots or lines and/or partial loss of vision; sensory symptoms such as numbness and/or pins and needles; and/or speech disturbance	On the same side as the headache: • red and/or watery eye • nasal congestion and/or runny nose • swollen eyelid • forehead and facial sweating • constricted pupil and/or drooping eyelid
Duration of headache	30 minutes to continuous	4 to 72 hours in adults 1 to 72 hours in young people aged 12 to 17 years	15 to 180 minutes

Figure 13.4   Distinguishing features between various primary headache disorders.

4. IMPORTANT CLINICAL POINTS FOR DIAGNOSIS OF MIGRAINE AND OTHER HEADACHES

a. In any patient with headache, a diagnosis of ***probable migraine*** is much more likely than a diagnosis of TTH. Probable migraine means, when a patient clinically fulfills either the pain criteria or the associated symptoms criteria, but not both.

b. There are 5 phases of migraine headache:
   i. Prodromal phase: Fatigue, impaired concentration, neck stiffness, food craving, irritability, mood changes.
   ii. Aura.
   iii. Headache.
   iv. Postdrome: 24–48 hours after headache: 80% have tiredness or weariness.
   v. Interictal phase.

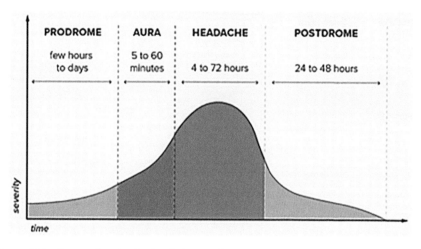

Figure 13.5   Phases of a migraine headache attack.

Migraine with AURA		
Auras are • Fully reversible symptoms • Develop gradually over 5 minutes • Last for 5–60 minutes	**Typical** aura symptoms • Visual: Flickering lights, spots • Negative: Partial loss of vision • Sensory: +/– Sensory symptoms • Speech changes	**Atypical aura: Investigate or refer to a specialist if** • Double vision • Loss of vision only one eye • Motor weakness • Poor balance • Loss of consciousness

   c. Premonitory symptoms of migraine can include neck stiffness but not hearing loss. So, any patient with hearing loss, be careful not to diagnose as migraine.

   d. Nausea and vomiting in migraine are localized to: **Dorsal medulla**.

Important points about migraine medications	
1. Triptans	**Naratriptan and Frovatriptan (6–26 hours)** Have longer t1/2 than other triptans (2–4 hours) All triptans are 5HT-1b agonists so they have vascular side effects Hence triptans should be used cautiously or avoided in patients: • Elderly • Coronary artery disease • Cerebrovascular disease
2. Ergots	**DHE nasal** spray: Preferred for migraine with **allodynia**
3. Propranolol	Worsens asthma, depression, diabetic status Before prescribing beta-blockers, always ask for history of asthma and diabetes. Beta-blockers are also known to cause generalized apathy and erectile dysfunction So, can be avoided in young and middle-aged men
4. Lasmiditan	**5HT-1f agonist:** Better than triptans—because no vascular side effects but impaired **driving x 8 hours** In many studies, Lasmiditan has been shown to be associated with impaired simulated driving performance at 1.5 hr post-dose

Important points about migraine medications	
5. CGRP antagonists	–gepants: Only 2 approved • Rimegepant: Orally available disintegrating tab • Ubrogepant: Repeat dosing required
6. CGRP monoclonal antibodies	Erenumab: CONSTIPATION is a major side effect
7. Sphenopalatine ganglion mediators	Molecules: CGRP, pituitary Adenyl Cyclase, VIP, NO
8. BotoxA	OnabotulinumtoxinA injections are a well-supported and well-established treatment option for chronic migraine and less so for other chronic headache disorders. The **tolerability of this approach compares** very favorably to oral medication since its local administration is associated with fewer systemic side effects

e. Migraine and women
    i. In pregnancy, migraine is least in 3rd trimester.
    ii. Headache is stable and is due to high Estrogen levels (and progesterone).
    iii. Migraine with aura is associated with higher risk of vascular disease: Pre-eclampsia
    iv. Menstrual headache: Start Frovatriptan 2 days prior; BD dose × 5 days.

f. Childhood migraine
    i. If onset <6 years: Will need preventive Rx.
    ii. If menarche attained <12 years: Increased odds of migraine.
    iii. Ibuprofen: 7.5–10 mg/kg 1st choice medication.
    iv. Rizatriptan 2nd choice.

g. Trigger point injections: Can be given in TTH.

h. **Hypnic headache** is a unique type of headache disorder in which daily **caffeine consumption** can result in improvement in headache. Daily caffeine intake in other headache disorders may cause exacerbation of headache or no benefit.

i. **Mental neuropathy**: Mandibular or meningeal metastasis from **Breast cancer.**

j. **Occipital neuralgia**: Pain starts over back of head and radiates to top of head: Rx: Physical therapy; TCAs, anti-seizure drugs, ON block, Botox.

k. Important clinical and diagnostic points about SIH (spontaneous intracranial hypotension).
    i. Patients who develop secondary complications of SIH, such as CVT **or subdural hematoma**, can have a change in their headache pattern with disappearance of the postural component or even development of a paradoxical postural aspect in which the headache worsens with lying.
    ii. The **venous distension sign of the dominant transverse** sinus has a high sensitivity and specificity for SIH.
    iii. Diffuse pachymeningeal enhancement is a classic sign of SIH, occurring because of pachymeningeal venous dilation and increased contrast transit time.
    iv. D/D of pachymeningeal enhancement: In other diseases; usually more **nodular or localized** than what is seen in spontaneous intracranial hypotension.
    v. Degree of **superior ophthalmic vein collapse** has been shown to correlate with intracranial pressures, with resolution of collapse noted after treatment of SIH.
    vi. Pituitary gland enlargement and **pituitary hyperemia** can be seen patients with SIH, but are not highly specific or sensitive findings.
    vii. Closure of the midbrain-pons angle is associated with a **suboptimal response** to at least a first attempt at epidural blood patch.
    viii. Slow leaks: Require radionucleotide scinitigraphy.

5. NICE GUIDELINES: HEADACHE

1.			Neuroimaging	Don't do imaging in patients with primary headache disorders like migraine/TTH/CH or MOH
2.			Counselling includes	Positive diagnosis and options of management Fact that headache is a disease which affects Quality of life Should be done in all patients
MIGRAINE				
3.			Acute Rx options In an acute attack of migraine:	• Oral triptan + NSAID • Oral triptan + PCM • Nasal (sumatriptan) triptan in <18 years (12–17 years)
			If not controlled by oral medicines	Try Non-oral metoclopramide or prochlorperazine Can add non-oral NSAID or triptan E.g.: Buccal prochlorperazine, nasal triptan
4.			Prophylactic therapy	Offer topiramate or propranolol • Propranolol: Increased harm in **depression** • Topiramate: Teratogenic Problems with topiramate • Cannot use in pregnancy • Reduced efficacy of hormonal contraceptives • So advise to use: Additional IUCD (intra-uterine contraceptive) or • Hormonal preparations + barrier or Medroxy progesterone acetate injection Amitriptyline: Evidence is limited—Randomized trial against Topiramate done, but no randomized trial against placebo Similarly; no good randomized trial for pizotifen **NO gabapentin** for prophylaxis **NO combined** hormonal contraceptives If topiramate or amitriptyline ineffective: Acupuncture 10 sessions (5–8 weeks) Riboflavin 400 mg OD may be used too Consider continuing treatment for 6 months
Menstrual migraine				For headaches that do not respond to standard treatment: Use Frovatriptan **(2.5 mg BD) or** Zolmitriptan **(2.5 mg BD-TDS)** on days migraine is expected

Pregnancy migraine		Acute Rx: PCM (Paracetamol) Consider use of NSAID or triptan Specialist referral for prophylactic treatment should be done	
5. CH (CLUSTER HEADACHE)			
a.		Acute Rx	Discuss the need of CT/MRI in 1st episode CH in consultation with specialist/neurophysician For Rx: Use Oxygen + subcutaneous or nasal triptan 100% @ >12 L/min in non-re-breathing mask + reservoir Arrange ambulatory + home oxygen NO NSAIDs NO triptans NO opioids, ergots in acute CH
b.		Triptans	Nasal triptans: NOT approved in CH Subcutaneous triptans: OFF label indication in CH, under-18 years
c.		Nasal triptans	Ensure optimal dose available as per clusters, based on manufacturer's maximum dose
d.		Prophylactic Rx for CH	Verapamil Consider specialist reference for using verapamil ECG monitoring is required Specialist referral if there is no response to verapamil Specialist referral if CH occurs in pregnancy
Absolute **NO Aspirin <16**: Aspirin can cause REYES syndrome in pediatric population.			

6. TTH: NO OPIOIDS FOR TTH (TENSION-TYPE HEADACHE)		
Consider 10 sessions of Acupuncture over a course of 5–8 weeks for chronic TTH How to differentiate CH from acute glaucoma? **Check pupils:** Constricted pupil in CH and semi-dilated in acute red eye glaucoma		
7. MOH (MEDICATION OVERUSE HEADACHE)		
	Stop all drugs **abruptly** Stop all drugs **x 1 month**	Abruptly stopping may increase headache in short term May have withdrawal symptoms But this will gradually improve Consider some other prophylactic Rx for underlying headache Review after 4–8 weeks Consider admission and In-patient withdrawal of drugs if • Patient is using strong opioids • Relevant comorbidities warrant admission • In whom previous repeated attempts at withdrawal were unsuccessful

(Continued)

(Continued)

8.	Consider further Investigation or referral for patients who have red flags Figure 13.6 Red flags.	Headache + fever Thunderclap headache (maximum intensity within 5 minutes) New-onset FND (focal neurological deficit) New-onset cognitive change Impaired consciousness Changed personality Recent head trauma (3 months) Headache triggered by **exercise** Headache triggered by cough, Valsalva Orthostatic headache Acute narrow angle glaucoma Giant cell arteritis Substantial change in character of headache
9.	Consider referral if	Immuno-compromised patient (HIV+/taking immunosuppressive drugs) Age <20 years + malignancy Malignancy which can metastasize into brain Vomiting without any obvious cause
10.	Headache diary should be maintained	For at least **8 weeks** Frequency, duration or severity of symptoms should be noted Associated symptoms to be noted Possible precipitants All prescribed OTC (over-the-counter drugs) Relation to menstruation also to be written

MOVEMENT DISORDERS

Abbreviations

- *AD*: Autosomal dominant
- *AR*: Autosomal recessive
- *APLA*: Anti-phospholipid syndrome
- *ARF*: Acute Rheumatic fever
- *CBD*: Cortico-basal degeneration
- *CJD*: Creutzfeldt–Jakob disease
- *CPK*: Serum creatinine phosphokinase levels
- *MCP*: Middle cerebellar peduncle
- *MDS*: Movement disorders
- *MSA*: Multisystem atrophy
- *NBIA*: Neurodegeneration with brain iron accumulation
- *OCP*: Oral contraceptive pills
- *PD*: Parkinsonism
- *SLE*: Systemic lupus erythematosus
- *UMN*: Upper motor neuron syndrome
- *VSNG*: Vertical supranuclear gaze palsy
- *w/o*: Without

1. CONGENITAL MDS: CHOREA SYNDROMES (CAUDATE ATROPHY)

	Disease	C/F	Clues to diagnosis
1.	ChA Chorea-acanthocytosis	Autosomal recessive disorder with • Chorea + • **Orofacial-lingual** dystonia • **Feeding dystonia**—tongue protrusion after contact with food • Frontal dysfunction • Sexual dis-inhibition • Seizures • Parkinsonism • Sensory Axonal neuropathy	Tongue dystonia Lower **lip bite** Neuropathy CPK ~500 MRI: Caudate atrophy Gene: VPS13a

(Continued)

(Continued)

	Disease	C/F	Clues to diagnosis
1.	ChA Chorea- acanthocytosis (Contd)	Mnemonic: "**Korea SOFA costs 500**" **Korea** = Choreo-acanthocytosis **S** = Sensory axonal neuropathy, seizures, sexual disinhibition **O** = Orofacial + lip biting dyskinesia **F** = Feeding dystonia **A** = Axonopathy + acanthocytosis **Costs** = CPK levels = ~500 Figure 14.1 Peripheral blood film showing acanthocytes.	

2.	HD
	Huntington
	disease
		Most common answer to any
		  question about chorea
		  • Even if no family history
		Sometimes parents die before
		being symptomatic
		  • So family history may be
		    absent
		  • (See in the question: If any
		    death around 50–60 years in a
		    family member)
		Clinical presentation: Chorea
		  • Semi-purposeful
		  • Irregular, jerky movements
		  • Flitting from one part to
		    another
		
		Autosomal dominant disorder due
		to
		  • Chromosome 4p—CAG repeats
		  • <26 repeats: Normal
		Instability in sperm is more than
		egg
		So, if father has HD—children have
		  much more CAGs
		
		Pre-manifest stage: 4S
		  • Slow saccades
		  • Slow EOM
		  • Slow finger tap
		  • Subtle frontal signs
		    • Stimulus sensitive myoclonus
		    • Suicidal tendency is 6x times
		      more
			
			Figure 14.2 MRI coronal showing caudate atrophy with boxcar ventricles.

	Disease	C/F	Clues to diagnosis
3.	Wilson Disease	Hepato-lenticular degeneration Deposition of copper leading to • Mixed movement disorders • Early prominent axial MDS • Wing beating tremors • WD facies and KF ring • Sunflower cataract Psychiatric MDS ◇ Liver Osseo-muscular Figure 14.3 • Cognitive—frontal dysfunction • Hyper-sexuality, touches inappropriately • Mischief at home, smokes inappropriately • Liver involved in 1st decade • Osseous features: Fleeting pains Blood tests • Low ceruloplasmin: 5% patients can have normal levels • High 24-h urinary copper • High liver biopsy copper • False high ceruloplasmin in cholestasis Rx: Zinc DOC, d-penicillamine, trientene, Ammonium TTH, BAL	AR ATP 7b Chromosome 13 Large gene: >600 mutation MRI: Bilateral T2 hyperintensity in putamen, thalami, Brainstem Signs • Double panda • Face of giant panda: Midbrain • Cub panda in pons

2. CHOREA GRAVIDARUM

BOX 14.1   CAUSES OF CHOREA GRAVIDARUM

- MCC: Rheumatic fever
- APLA
- SLE
- Wilson disease
- Huntington disease
- Thyrotoxicosis

a. Rare disorder.
b. Usually occurs in 1st Trimester.
c. Remission seen in 3rd Trimester in 33% patients.
d. Remission after delivery seen in 100% patients.
e. Patients are prone to recurrence in next pregnancy.
f. They are also prone to recurrence with use of OCP.
g. Most patients have a recurrence in subsequent pregnancies.

h. Most common Risk Factor: ARF.

i. Cause of chorea gravidarum: Hormonal imbalances in pregnancy.

j. Thyrotoxicosis is commonly associated with CG (not hypothyroidism).

3. CONGENITAL MDS: NBIA (GLOBUS PALLIDUS AND THALAMUS INVOLVEMENT)

a. All NBIAs are autosomal recessive, except:
- Neuroferritinopathy (Autosomal dominant).
- MPAN (Autosomal dominant or Autosomal recessive).
- BPAN (X-linked).

	Disease	Clinical features	Diagnosis
1.	PKAN (PANK2) Pantothenate Kinase-Associated Neurodegeneration	Early onset ~3 years Late onset >10 years Onset with GAIT abnormality @3 years • + Parkinsonism • + DYSARTHRIA • + Retinal degeneration/ pigmentosa • UMN signs (spasticity, Babinski sign) Figure 14.4 Axial T2-MRI showing eye of the tiger sign.	Eye of tiger sign • Coronal or axial section MRI • GP nucleus shows a • Central hyperintensity with a surrounding hypointensity
		Spank the tiger: Eye + speech + walking (3 signs @ 3 yrs) gives the eye of tiger!!	
2.	PLAN- PLA2g6-associated neurodegeneration PARK-9	Dystonia–parkinsonism syndrome • Infantile onset • Juvenile onset • Adult onset Milestone regression + Dystonia + Parkinsonism + UMN + Gait abnormality	Genetic tests help in diagnosis
3.	KRS Kufor–Rakeb syndrome PARK-9	Rare inherited parkinsonism syndrome Hallmark features are • Vertical SN gaze palsy • Facial-faucial-finger myoclonus	Genetic tests help in diagnosis

	Disease	Clinical features	Diagnosis
4.	Neuro-ferritinopathy	Similar to Huntington Disease, but there are Prominent orofacial action dystonia Belongs to the group of HD phenocopy disease	HD phenocopy diseases are usually autosomal dominant diseases
5.	BPAN Beta-propeller protein-associated neurodegeneration	X-linked disease characterized by • Childhood seizures + • Dystonia-parkinsonism-dementia	
6.	FAHN Fatty Acid Hydroxylase-associated Neurodegeneration	A-T-S-O • Ataxia • Tetraparesis • Seizures • Optic atrophy May start with leg dystonias	Classified under NBIA and also under leukodystrophy
7.	Aceruloplasminemia	Usually presents in adults: 20–60 years The clinical triad is shown Figure 14.5. There is also Anemia + iron overload + Diabetes mellitus **High ferritin, near absent ceruloplasmin**** Low iron, Copper levels Facial-neck dystonia—blepharospasm Cervical dystonia Facial grimacing	Treatment: Iron chelation Retinal degeneration DM ⟋⟍ Neuro disorder Figure 14.5 Triad of aceruloplasminemia.
		MRI: GRE or SWI images will show Iron deposition in Basal ganglia • Globus pallidus • Thalamus • Substantia Nigra • Red Nucleus • Dentate nucleus Figure 14.6 MRI axial images showing iron deposition in dentate nucleus, substantia nigra and bilateral basal ganglia.	
8.	WSS Woodhouse–Sakati syndrome	Childhood onset A-D-H-M **A**lopecia + **D**iabetes mellitus + **H**ypogonadism + **M**ental retardation	

4. IDIOPATHIC (LATE-ONSET) MOVEMENT DISORDERS WHICH MAY OR MAY NOT AFFECT COGNITION

	Disease	Clinical features	Diagnosis
1.	Parkinson's disease	The cardinal features are • Bradykinesia • Rigidity • Tremors • Postural instability • Asymmetric or unilateral onset	Diagnosis is made by the UK–Brain Bank criteria Brain Bank criteria specificity: 80–90% DOPA-PET scan may also be used in diagnosis
	Latest Treatment	Apomorphine: Onset of action is in 7–10 minutes • Duration of action: 45–60 minutes • Intermittent subcutaneous injections • Used as a Rescue therapy for on/off states	
2.	MSA Multisystem atrophy	Usually, bilateral symmetrical Laryngeal dystonia Autonomic—incontinence Sleep disorders **Polyminimyoclonus**** stimulus sensitive and Increases during voluntary movements	**MSA-P**: Putaminal atrophy Putaminal hyperintensity in Postero-lateral putamen **MSA-C**: Hot cross bun sign MCP hyperintensity Hot cross bun is seen in very few cases of MSA-C
		D/D laryngeal dystonia • MSA • DYT 2,5 (oro-mandibular) • DYT 4 (whispering) • KRS (finger-faucial-facial) myoclonus **D/D Hot cross bun sign** • MSA- C • Spinocerebellar ataxia • Autoimmune/para-neoplastic rhombencephalitis • Stroke • Vasculitis • Neurosarcoidosis • CBD, vCJD	
3.	Perry Syndrome	Rapidly progressive Parkinsonism **+ Apathy/depression** **+ Central hypoventilation** (late symptom) Onset ~50 years (47 years) Parkinsonism is mild BUT Depression is severe Suicidal tendencies ++ Father h/o suicide Vertical gaze palsy ~PSP	Psychiatric PD ◇ Weight loss Slow breathing **Figure 14.7** Features of Perry syndrome. DCTN-1 Dynactin mutation Autosomal dominant
4.	PSP Progressive supranuclear palsy	Parkinsonism + Vertical supranuclear gaze palsy Procerus sign Dementia Rocket sign	MRI brain named signs • Penguins and hummingbirds of midbrain atrophy

	Disease	Clinical features	Diagnosis
5.	CBD Cortico-basal degeneration	Asymmetric, Unilateral disease Limb apraxia Alien limb phenomenon Falls, postural instability is seen **Cortical sensory** and speech defects Difficulty **initiating saccades*** Most Common feature: Rigidity (90%) Least common: Myoclonus (20%)	Armstrong criteria used for diagnosis
6.	FTD Fronto-temporal dementia	Parkinsonism Dementia Mainly frontal and temporal dysfunction	Peri-sylvian atrophy seen on MRI Knife edge atrophy of frontal and temporal lobes
7.	PP-AOG Primary progressive apraxia of gait	Freezing of gait Difficulty gait initiation Festination Repetitive finger movements Tachyphemia (speech) W/o VSNG palsy, w/o rigidity, w/o tremors	Most have PSP pathology Less common: Lewy body pathology

5. DRUG-INDUCED MDS

	Disease	C/F	Diagnosis and Rx
1.	Drug-induced action tremors	Onset of tremors after drug initiation Worsening of tremors if dose increased Resolution of tremor if dose decreased or stopped Bilateral hand action tremor • *Head tremor is not a C/F of drug-induced tremor • *Head tremor is seen in Essential tremor or Cerebellar tremors	Sodium valproate–induced tremors are most common seen clinically Usually resolve once the drug is stopped.
2.	Drug-induced parkinsonism	Common clinical scenario: A previously epileptic patient has started to slow down in activities of daily living	Sodium Valproate (5%): Most common cause Ioflupane SPECT: Normal uptake Treatment is stopping the drug. Can use Levodopa or Trihexyphenidyl

(Continued)

(Continued)

	Disease	C/F	Diagnosis and Rx
3.	Edentulous oro-dyskinesia	H/o multiple tooth extraction Orofacial dyskinesia, chewing movements + Repetitive stereotype movements of jaw No tongue movements D/t loss of proprioception D/B: Tardive dyskinesia—No **tongue movements** in edentulous, prominent in TD	
4.	Tardive dyskinesia	Prominent abnormal tongue movements Like: Chewing, lip smacking Cause: Dopamine blockers	Rx • Tetrabenazine >> THP, amantadine When withdrawal of drug not possible (psychiatric or schizophrenia): Better to use • Clozapine: Minimum risk** • 2nd choice: Quetiapine • 3rd choice: Aripiperazole Pharmacogenetics: CYP 2D6: Tetrabenazine inefficient metabolizers

6. TREMORS

	Disease	C/F	Diagnosis and Rx
1.	Holmes tremors/ Rubral tremor/ Midbrain tremor	Rubral tremor are • Slow tremors, <4.5 Hz • Combination of Rest + postural + action tremor • Cause: Ischemia or hemorrhage in the Midbrain, thalamus or cerebellum	Levodopa may help in 50% Functional surgery (DBS)
2.	EPT Enhanced physiological tremor	Low-amplitude tremor High-frequency tremor Both hands are involved All fingers symmetrically Very little or no intentional component Occurs primarily when a posture is maintained Cause: Stress, anxiety, drugs, toxins, Thyroxine, caffeine Most common cause of postural tremor	Rx: Identification and removal or treatment of the precipitating cause such as: • Thyrotoxicosis • Hypoglycemia • Emotional stress • Pheochromocytoma Drugs used: Tricyclic antidepressants, neuroleptics and lithium

	Disease	C/F	Diagnosis and Rx
3.	ET Essential tremor	Clear intentional component **Intentional*** more prominent than postural tremor Unidirectional tremor Unidirectional axis Flexion-extension of wrist Depends on the hand used Commonly 8 o'clock–2 o'clock direction for right hand and 10 o'clock–4 o'clock for left hand SCA-12 can mimic ET	Genetic factors Autosomal dominant Positive family history Should do a genetic analysis to rule out SCA-12 Drugs used: • Beta-blockers • Primidone
4.	Vocal/Laryngeal tremors	Mostly seen with • ET • PD • Spasmodic dysphonia • Very rarely with EPT	
5.	Head tremors	**Not a feature of EPT May be seen in cerebellar tremor or ET	
6.	Orthostatic tremor	• Subjective unsteadiness on standing • Relieved on sitting • Relieved on walking May rarely be a.w.: • PD • DLBD • PSP • Vascular Parkinsonism	EMG: 13–18 Hz tremor while standing Rx: Clonazepam > beta-blockers

PD tremor	ET tremor	EPT
Asymmetric Rest tremor	Symmetric Postural tremor	Symmetric Variable
High amplitude	Mid-amplitude	Low amplitude
Low frequency 4–6 Hz	Mid-frequency 5–8 Hz	High frequency 8–12 Hz
Only rest tremor May have re-emergent tremor	No other neuro deficits Resolves with Alcohol	Increased by stress and coffee

7. DYSKINESIA

a. All are AD (autosomal dominant) and more common in males, except PED
   i. NK—starts early, <5 years, but has prolonged attacks (up to hours).
   ii. PKD—starts later: 5–15 years, but has shorter attacks (<5 minutes).
   iii. PED starts after 20 years, with 20 minute attacks, and is due to exercise, coffee and alcohol.

	Disease	C/F	Diagnosis
1.	Functional dyskinesias	Sudden movements Figure 14.8 Bereitschaftspotential.	Bereit-schafts-potentials = Pre-motor potential = Readiness potentials Activity in motor cortex
2.	PNKD Paroxysmal non-kinesiogenic dyskinesia	Onset <5 years Duration: Minutes to hours 2 times/day to 2 times/year: Attack frequency Patient reports "spasms in UL/LL" Aura: Preceded by feeling of "tightness" Exacerbated by **alcohol, caffeine**, excitement Rx: Clonazepam, oxazepam	Associated with • MR-1 gene • Ataxia, chorea
3.	PKD Paroxysmal kinesiogenic dyskinesia	Onset: 5–15 years age Short attacks: <5 minute attack More in frequency: Can be 10–100 per day Exacerbated by: **Sudden movement**, stress, fatigue Hyperventilation Rx: PHT (phenytoin), CBZ (carbamazepine), BZD (benzodiazepine)	PRRT-2 gene Epilepsy, chorea
		Remember, PKD—associated with epilepsy— Attacks also like epilepsy—short and more frequent Treatment also with antiepileptic drugs	
4.	PED Paroxysmal exercise–induced dyskinesia	Onset >20 years Attacks longer: 20 minutes More in females 1 per/day to 1 per/month	GLUT gene SLCA-2A1
5	EA-2 Episodic ataxia-2	Onset <20 years Autosomal dominant Attacks of BAV (balance/ataxia/vertigo) Imbalance + ataxia + vertigo Precipitated by stress, anxiety, alcohol, caffeine Interictal nystagmus may be seen	CACNA1A P/Q type—Purkinje cells 50% have migraine MRI: Mild vermis (midline) atrophy Rx: Acetazolamide
	EA-4	~EA-2, interictal nystagmus Onset >20 years No response to Acetazolamide	
	EA-5	~EA-2	CACNB4

	Interictal	Gene	Chromosome 19 CACN a1 ds:
EA-1	Myokymia, neuromyotonia	KCN a1	
EA-2	Nystagmus, migraine	CACN a1	**FHM-1**
EA-3	Tinnitus		**EA-2**
EA-4	Nystagmus (>20 years)		**SCA-6**
EA-5	Nystagmus	CACN b4	
EA-6	Alternating hemiplegia	SLC 1a3	

8. STIFF PERSON SYNDROME (SPS)

a. Rare disease.
b. Fluctuating rigidity and stiffness.
c. Axial and proximal limb muscles.
d. Painful spasms in neck, back.
e. Unable to bend over.
f. Adopts a hyperlordotic posture.
g. Spasms provoked by anxiety, sudden noise, movement.
h. EMG: Continuous contraction of agonists, antagonists.
i. Abdomen and paraspinal muscles.
j. Serum may have GAD antibodies.
k. SPS and Diabetes mellitus co-exist in 35% patients.

Type of attack	Clinical correlation
Episodic very short spasms with movement	PPRT-PKD: Rx with CBZ, PHT
Episodic medium lasting spasms with alcohol and caffeine in child	MR-PNKD
Episodic back and neck spasms, fluctuating	SPS

9. CHILDHOOD ATAXIC DISORDERS

	Disease	C/F	Diagnostic clues and Rx
1.	ARSACS Autosomal recessive spastic ataxia of Charlevoix–Saguenay Mnemonic: **5S-M**	Seen in Quebec, Canada Childhood-onset gait ataxia + • *Spastic ataxia: Spasticity + • Distal *Muscle wasting • Bidirectional nystagmus + • *Saccadic alteration of *Smooth pursuits • *Saccadic dysmetria • *Superior cerebellum vermis atrophy Late involvement of cerebellar hemisphere, Spinal cord	AR **S**ACS3 gene **NCS**: Initial demyelination seen Later axonal neuropathy MVP (mitral valve prolapse) occurs in 50%
2.	CoQ deficiency ataxia	Ataxia + spasticity + seizures	
3.	Refsum disease	Ataxia + Retinitis Pigmentosa + SNHL (hearing loss) + Peripheral Neuropathy + cataract	
4.	Naito-Oyanagi disease: DRPLA Dentatorubral-Pallidoluysian atrophy Mnemonic: MEADC	**M**yoclonus + **E**pilepsy + **A**taxia + **C**ognitive **D**ecline (decline in cognitive ability) Onset: ~30 years Juvenile: <20 years: Have more myoclonic epilepsy Adult: >20 years: More chorea + cerebellar ataxia C/P depends on age and the number of CAG repeats Anticipation ++ So, father will have onset in 30s-40s, but children will have it a decade earlier—in 20s <20 years: Seizures common 20–40: Seizures less common >40 years: Seizures not seen (also CAG <65)	Asian** CAG repeats DrpLA gene—atrophin protein Anticipation **M-E-A-D-C** (chorea) MRI atrophy • Brainstem • Cerebellum • Pons tegmentum

10. ATAXIA IN ELDERLY

	Disease	C/F	Diagnosis
1.	DRPLA Dentatorubral-Pallidoluysian atrophy	In elderly—seizures are not seen Only **ADS** out of MEADS remains • **A**taxia • **D**ementia (cognitive decline) • **S**pasticity; choreo-athetoid movements Myoclonus and epilepsy (M/E of MEADS) seen in children	AD, DRPLA aTrophin protein
2.	Superficial siderosis	Past h/o intra-dural or cranial or spinal surgery Onset with sub-acute ataxia + dysarthria + Bilateral hearing loss: SNHL + Spasticity and weakness Hemosiderin deposit seen in sub-pial layers Source of bleeding is • CNS vascular tumours (ependymoma) • CNS cavity lesions (meningocele, myelocele, ncephalo-pseudomeningocele)	MRI T2: **Hypointensity along the contours** of brain/Spinal cord SWI blooming due to hemosiderin
3.	FXTAS Fragile X-tremor ataxia syndrome	7th decade onset Tremors Ataxia	55–200 CGG repeats Bilateral MCP sign
4.	Opsoclonus myoclonus syndrome	Para-neoplastic disorder No CSF antibody currently described Other causes • Post-COVID demyelination • 2–3 weeks after COVID infection May be seen in certain other viral infections	

11. COVID-INDUCED MOVEMENT DISORDERS

a. Although COVID has been associated with hypercoagulability and strokes, some movement disorders have also been reported.

b. COVID-induced tic disorders = Functional neurological disorders.

c. COVID-induced opsoclonus myoclonus.

12. PONS AND CEREBELLAR RADIOLOGICAL SIGNS IN MDS

	Sign	D/D
1.	**Hot cross bun sign**	MSA-C Spinocerebellar ataxia Autoimmune/para-neoplastic rhombencephalitis Stroke Vasculitis Neurosarcoidosis CBD, vCJD

	Sign	D/D
2.	MCP hyperintensities seen in middle cerebellar peduncle (main afferent to cerebellum) Figure 14.9	SCA MSA-C FXTAS Wilson Hypoglycemia Toluene toxicity EPM PML AICA infarct or Wallerian degeneration (unilateral) U/L: Demyelination of axons: MS Neurodegeneration: Preferential loss of Purkinje cells and GM nuclei Axonal loss and loss of MCP Neoplastic process is rare
3.	123-I-Ioflupane DAT scan	
	Bilateral "Comma-shaped" basal ganglia	Normal or • Drug-induced PD • Dopa-responsive Dystonia
	Asymmetric scan	PD PSP
	Symmetric abnormal	Vascular PD if Basal ganglia infarcts
	Absent in putamen but + in caudate	
	Absent in both caudate and putamen	

Example of normal DaTscan image

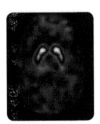

In transaxial images, normal images are characterized by two symmetric comma- or crescent-shaped focal regions of activity mirrored about the median plane. Striatal activity is distinct, relative to surrounding brain tissue

Examples of abnormal DaTscan images :

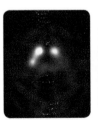

Activity is asymmetric, eg, activity in the region of the putamen of one hemisphere is absent or greatly reduced with respect to the other. Activity is still visible in the caudate nuclei of both hemispheres, resulting in a comma or crescent shape in one and a circular or oval focus in the other. There may be reduced activity between at least one striatum and surrounding tissues

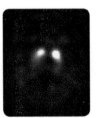

Activity is absent in the putamen of both hemispheres and confined to the caudate nuclei. Activity is relatively symmetric and forms two roughly circular or oval foci. Activity of one or both is generally reduced

Activity is absent in the putamen of both hemispheres and greatly reduced in one or both caudate nuclei. Activity of the striata with respect to the background is reduced

Figure 14.10

13. MISCELLANEOUS QUESTIONS

a. Tourette syndrome: MC a.w. ADHD and OCD.

b. >1 Vocal/motor tic >1 year: A diagnosis of Tourette disorder is made when the person has two or more motor tics and at least one vocal tic—even if these do not happen at the same time. Tics must persist for more than one year.

c. Dystonia + myoclonus: DYT 11: Epsilon-SCG: SCGE.

d. Suppose a patient on newer anticoagulants (NOAC/DOAC) has to undergo any procedure—When to stop DOAC

    i. Apixaban and rivaroxaban 24 hours.

    ii. Dabigatran stopped 48 hours.

    iii. Re-introduced 6 hours after surgery.

14. NICE GUIDELINES: PARKINSON'S DISEASE (PD)

a. Levodopa: 1st line for PD patients whose motor symptoms affect QoL (quality of life).

b. PD + hallucinations/delusions, but no cognitive decline (see MMSE/MoCA).

    i. Drug of choice: Quetiapine.

    ii. 2nd line choice: Clozapine.

    iii. Olanzapine is not recommended.

c. PD-dementia + hallucinations: Some evidence that rivastigmine helps.

Parkinson's disease category	NICE guideline recommendations
Suspect PD when patient has	Tremor + slowness of activities Stiffness, gait problems Difficulty walking
What to do	When suspected—refer to specialist
Diagnosis of Parkinson's disease	As per the UK Brain Bank criteria At the time of diagnosis: Encourage the patient to donate tissue to brain bank
Review diagnosis	Review diagnosis every 6–12 months See if any atypical features develop • This is important for early identification of Parkinson-plus syndromes
SPECT (123-I-FP-CIT)	Should be available to specialist Done if we cannot differentiate between ET and PD tremor
DO NOT USE	Structural MRI to diagnose PD MRI volumetry PET scan in differential diagnosis of PD, except in trials MRS (MR spectroscopy) Levodopa challenge test Apomorphine challenge test Objective smell testing
DO NOT use these modalities in differential diagnosis of atypical PD	MRS (MR spectroscopy) PET scan Levodopa challenge Apomorphine challenge Objective smell testing
Can be used in trials	Objective smell test MRS (MR spectroscopy) PET scan
Can be used for differential diagnosis of atypical PD	Structural MRI

Parkinson's disease category	NICE guideline recommendations

	LEVODOPA	DOPA AGONISTS	MAO-B INHIBITORS
MOTOR symptoms	More improvement	Less improvement	Less improvement
Activities of daily living	More improvement in ADLS	Less improvement	Less improvement
Motor complications	More motor complications	Less	Less
Adverse events Excessive sleepiness Hallucinations Impulse control disorders	Fewer specific adverse events	More	Fewer specified adverse events

Figure 14.11

NO role of (in Rx of PD)	Drug holidays Drug abrupt withdrawal See for malabsorption (diarrhea, surgery) in case of no clinical effect
1st line Rx (early PD)	Motor symptoms affect QoL: Start Levodopa Motor symptoms do not affect QoL: Dopamine agonist, Levodopa or MAO-B **NO role of ergots***
Discuss and record	ICD (impulse control disorder) with dopaminergic therapy Excessive sleepiness and sudden-onset sleep with dopa agonists Psychotic sx (Delusion + Hallucination) with dopaminergic therapy
Dyskinesia or fluctuations with levodopa therapy	Offer add-ons as per Figure 14.12 Choice depends on patient's clinical condition, comorbidity etc. Choose a non-ergot-derived DA Monitoring is required with ergot-DA Hence, better NOT to use: Ergot DA, anticholinergics

	DOPA AGONISTS	MAO-B INHIBITORS	COMT INHIBITORS	AMANTADINE
MOTOR symptoms	Improvement in motor symptoms	Improvement	Improvement	No evidence of improvement
Activities of daily living	Improvement in ADLS	Improvement	Improvement	No evidence of improvement
OFF time	More off-time reduction	Off-time reduction	Off-time reduction	No evidence
Adverse events Excessive sleepiness Hallucinations Impulse control disorders	Immediate risk of adverse events More hallucinations	Fewer adverse events Less hallucinations	More adverse events Less hallucinations	No studies reporting on these

Figure 14.12

(*Continued*)

(Continued)

Parkinson's disease category	NICE guideline recommendations
Dyskinesia, fluctuation during treatment	Choose a non-ergot-derived DA Only choose ergot DA if • Non-ergot-derived DA not able to control fluctuations/dyskinesia
If still not controlled	• Offer amantadine
ICD Impulse control disorder	Can develop on any therapy, at any time of PD Risk factors for ICD • Previous impulsive behavior • Previous alcohol or smoking • More risk with dopamine agonists
Examples of ICD	Compulsive gambling, binge eating, hypersexuality, obsessive shopping
Rx of ICD	Seek specialist help 1st consider reducing DA Offer cognitive behavior therapy
Daytime sleepiness	Inform DVLA Seek specialist help to adjust medicines Can offer modafinil if other causes ruled out Monitor and re-evaluate at every 12 months
RBD treatment	Clonazepam or melatonin
Nocturnal akinesia	Consider levodopa or DA If not successful—consider ROTIGOTINE
Orthostatic hypotension	Review these meds • Anti-HTN (diuretics) • Dopaminergics • Anticholinergics • Antidepressants Can offer: Midodrine If not tolerated or contraindication to midodrine: Fludrocortisone Cardiac risk is there with fludrocortisone
Delusion and hallucination	DO NOT Rx if well-tolerated Otherwise: Quetiapine >> clozapine **Doses required in PD are lower than usual psychotic doses**** No olanzapine No phenothiazines, butryphenones (worsen motor symptoms)
PD-dementia	Mild-moderate: Offer cholinesterase inhibitors Severe PDD: Consider cholinesterase inhibitors 2nd line: Memantine
Saliva drooling in PD patients	1st line: Speech and language therapy 2nd line: Glycopyrronium bromide But problem is: Delusion + Hallucination + cognitive abnormalities with this drug • In that case—botox can be offered
Neuroprotection	NO vitamin E NO CoQ NO DA NO MAO-B

Parkinson's disease category	NICE guideline recommendations
Physiotherapy role in PD	Start early in PD **ALEXANDER technique**** for motor and balance
Occupational therapy	Important in PD
Speech and language therapy	EMST (expiratory muscle strength training) Alternative and Augmentative communication equipment
Diet	Diet plan Most of the protein should be eaten in the last meal of the day **Protein re-distribution****: For fluctuations

NEURO-INFECTIONS

Abbreviations

- *C/F*: Clinical features
- *Dwi*: MRI diffusion-weighted
- *O/E*: On examination
- *MoCA*: Montreal Cognitive Assessment

1. CREUTZFELDT–JAKOB DISEASE (CJD)

	Disease	Clinical features	Diagnosis and radiology
1.	sCJD Sporadic Creutzfeldt– Jakob disease	sCJD is Extremely rare • Fatal • Neurodegenerative • Spongiform transmissible encephalopathy • Also called prion disease C/P: **Rapidly declining memory** (x 2–4 months) • With agitation, poor recall • Behavior changes • Personality changes • Sleeping difficulty O/E—Mild-to-moderate rigidity • Very low MoCA scores	MRI shows • Focal or diffuse • Symmetrical or asymmetric • Involvement of cortex and basal ganglia • Cerebellar atrophy Peri-Rolandic cortex is spared** Atypical features • Peri-Rolandic involvement • Hockey stick or pulvinar sign
	MRI-DWI is the most sensitive for diagnosis of early disease** CSF RT QuIC: Has 92% Sensitivity and 100% specificity **MRI-DWI: Cortical ribboning—Hyperintense signals in gyriform pattern** (see Figure 15.1) **FLAIR: Mild caudate/putamen hyperintensity** **Cortical + deep GM hyperintensities** 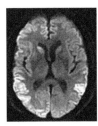 Figure 15.1 Axial DWI MRI images showing cortical ribboning.		

DOI: 10.1201/b23306-15

	Disease	Clinical features	Diagnosis and radiology
2.	vCJD Variant sporadic Creutzfeldt–Jakob disease Mnemonic **(PT–CAD)**	Early symptoms (PT) • **P**sychiatric symptoms • **T**halamic sensory loss Late symptoms (CAD) • **C**erebellar ataxia • **A**taxia • **D**ementia MRI: Hockey stick sign (thalamic involvement) Figure 15.2 Axial MRI FLAIR images showing pulvinar sign.	

Clinical features	sCJD	vCJD
Mean age of onset	65 years	29 years
Median duration of illness	4 months	14 months
Early symptoms	–	Psychiatric Thalamic
Dementia	Early	Late
Cerebellar ataxia	Early	Late
Thalamic pain symptoms	–	Early

2. BACTERIAL MENINGITIS AND ENCEPHALITIS

		Clinical	Radiology and diagnosis
MENINGITIS: TRIAD OF FEVER + HEADACHE + MENINGEAL SIGNS			
1.	HiB Hemophilus influenza B	Main risk factors • Children/Pediatric group • Splenectomy • Unimmunized children • 5% of all adult bacterial meningitis Diagnosis by: CSF studies • Increased CSF cell count	Gram stain Gram-Negative Coco-bacilli Figure 15.3　Gram-negative coco-bacilli.
2.	Strep **pn** *Streptococcus pneumoniae*	Main risk factors • Children/Pediatric group • Elderly • Most common causes of meningitis in both these age groups Facultative anerobic bacteria Alpha-hemolytic (in aerobic conditions) Beta-hemolytic (anerobic conditions)	Gram-Positive cocci (GPC) Diplococci Lancet-shaped Figure 15.4　Gram-positive diplococci.
3.	*Neisseria*	More common in infants and children <2 years Gonococcus Gram-Negative cocci (GNC)—diplococcus	 Figure 15.5　Gram-negative diplococci.

(Continued)

(Continued)

		Clinical	Radiology and diagnosis
4.	Listeria	Listeria **rhomben**cephalitis Listeria causes **Ponto-medullary** encephalitis May occur in immunocompetent or Immunocompromised host C/F • Prodromal phase for few days • Fever headache, Nausea, Vomiting • Followed by neurological signs • Diplopia, Lateral Rectus palsy • Dysarthria • Weakness, spasticity, brisk DTR	MRI shows T2 hyperintensities in • Brainstem • Cerebellum is less commonly involved • Upper Cervical spine may be involved CSF shows: Lymphocytosis + elevated protein
5.	WD Whipple disease	Caused by *Tropheryma whipplei* WD is a Multisystem disease Joint pains precede others C/P by years • Diarrhea • Malabsorption • CNS: Decreased consciousness • Rigidity, spasticity, myoclonus • **Vertical Supranuclear gaze palsy** • **Oculo-masticatory myorrhythmia** • **Oculo-facial-skeletal myo-rhythmia**	 Figure 15.6 PAS-positive macrophages in biopsy. MRI brain: Non-specific changes CSF: Elevated cells or protein (non-specific) CSF PCR + for Trophyrema Small bowel Biopsy: PAS + macrophages
		Differential diagnosis of causes of supranuclear gaze palsy a. PSP—progressive supranuclear gaze palsy b. Whipple disease c. NP-C: Niemann–Pick disease C	

3. VIRAL INFECTIONS OF THE NERVOUS SYSTEM

	Disease	Clinical features	Diagnosis and radiology
1.	HSV Herpes simplex encephalitis	Most common encephalitis** Most common sporadic encephalitis Most common **fatal sporadic** encephalitis Clinical triad of encephalitis Fever + Headache + confusion (seizures)	MRI shows: Involvement • Unilateral or Bilateral temporal lobes • Insular cortex • Angular gyrus
		MRI and CSF may be normal in first 48–72 hours Hence, clinical suspicion is very important Treatment of choice is Acyclovir Indications for **stopping acyclovir** • Alternate diagnosis is made • CSF- HSV is negative on 2 occasions, 24–48 hours apart + MRI is not suggestive of HSV • CSF-HSV is negative when tested after 72 hours along with Normal consciousness, normal MRI and CSF cell <5 Neurological relapse in HSV encephalitis (relapse within days or weeks) • Relapse is well-known in HSV encephalitis • May be due to viral illness relapse, or • Anti-NMDA-receptor encephalitis	
2.	NMDA encephalitis N-methyl D-aspartate (NMDA) receptor	Suspect in any recent patient of HSV encephalitis who has neuro deterioration, and • No evidence of CSF-HSV • No response to acyclovir **C/P** • **Children: Mainly movement** disorders • **Adults: Psychiatric**** disorder	CSF in HSV encephalitis **30% may show NMDA-receptor antibodies**
3.	KBS Klüver–Bucy syndrome	KBS is frequently seen in patients with HSV encephalitis C/P • Docile • Hyper-orality • Hyper-sexuality • Visual agnosia • Pelvic thrusting, rubbing • Decreased emotional reactions Other Causes of KBS • Trauma • FTD: Fronto-temporal dementia	MRI brain shows • Involvement of the Anterior or medial temporal lobe • Bilateral **amygdala damage****

(Continued)

(Continued)

	Disease	Clinical features	Diagnosis and radiology
4.	VZV Varicella zoster encephalitis	History of • Recent VZV—herpes zoster or varicella rash • Followed in few weeks or months by • Neurological symptoms • Infarctions or • Hemorrhage A combination of both infarctions and hemorrhage is due to = vascular involvement by VZV VZV can develop months after rash Or may have no rash at all Most common vascular involvement • Large + small arteries (50% cases) • Only small arteries (33% cases)	VZV **IgG in CSF = 90%** of cases Due to Intrathecal synthesis CSF VZV DNA seen in only 33% cases MRI shows • Multifocal • Infarctions and • Hemorrhage • Hemorrhage appear T1-hyperintense Rx: IV acyclovir + steroids
5.	SSPE Sub-acute sclerosing pan-encephalitis **Dawsons disease***	Progressive cognitive decline with Motor decline Myoclonus, and leads to Death within 1–3 years of onset • Mainly a childhood disease, • But adult cases have been reported • Most common C/P: MYOCLONUS** • Slow myoclonus • Visual deterioration	MRI: Non-specific findings CSF: High titre of IgG anti-measles Antibodies **Diagnosis is made by Dyken Criteria** **Rademecker and Cobb** and Hill complexes: • High voltage (100–1000 mV) • Repetitive • Polyphasic discharges • On a slow background
		EEG: Periodic complexes in 60–85% Stereotyped, bilateral synchronous, Symmetrical 100–1000 mV, 1–3 Hz slow waves (delta) Intermixed with sharp waves or spikes	
6.	Hepatitis-C	Most common cause of **Mixed cryo-globulinaemia** • Most common C/P: Peripheral neuropathy • May be sensory neuropathy or • Sensori-motor neuropathy or • Mononeuritis multiplex C/P • Fever, recurrent Pyrexia of Unknown origin • Arthralgias • Raynaud's phenomenon • Foot drop, dorsiflexion weakness • Reduced sensations in distal UL and LL • Glove and stocking distribution	**NCS: AXONAL** neuropathy **Hepatitis C antibodies are positive in serum**

	Disease	Clinical features	Diagnosis and radiology
7.	HAD HIV-associated Dementia/ Cognitive dysfunction	Changes in HIV may range from asymptomatic or Mild cognitive impairment to HAD HAD includes • Cognitive loss >2 SD below mean • In >2 cognitive domains • There may be Apathy • Psychomotor slowing	HAD incidence has reduced in era of ART (anti-retroviral therapy) Investigations: Low CD4 counts MRI: Symmetrical involvement • Patchy or confluent • Leukoencephalopathy • + Cerebral atrophy D/D: PML: Unilateral changes: **No atrophy** usually

C/P	HAD	PML
Clinical features	Diffuse, bilateral	Unilateral, focal deficits
Cause	HIV virus	JC virus
MRI-T1	Isointense	Hypointense
MRI contrast	No enhancement	Mild enhancement
NCCT	Isodense	Hypodense
Distribution	Bilateral, symmetrical	Unilateral, sub-cortical

	Disease	Clinical features	Diagnosis and radiology
8.	PML	Progressive and multifocal deficits In a patient of HIV Low CD4 counts Taking immunosuppressants • Multifocal deficits • Cognitive decline • Visuo-spatial symptoms • Motor symptoms—hemiparesis	MRI: Unilateral changes JC virus antibody Biopsy • **Giant astrocytes**** • Altered oligodendroglia • Nuclei containing viral particles • Myelin loss (demyelination)
		MRI shows Patchy Sub-cortical white matter disease • Asymmetrical • No edema • No enhancement on contrast • White matter lesions—mainly seen in • **Parieto-occipital** lobes	
9.	HIV-Myelopathy	HIV causes **VACUOLAR** myelopathy Most common cause of Spinal cord involvement in HIV-1 It has a sub-acute progression	MRI spine • Long segment hyperintensity ****Typically Spinal cord atrophy seen; No enhancement** ~Findings are similar as seen in HTLV

(Continued)

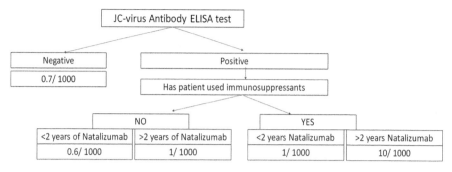

Figure 15.7 Estimating the risk of PML in a patient of HIV.

BOX 15.1   RISK OF PML IN A PATIENT OF HIV ON NATALIZUMAB

- 0.6–0.7/1000 if
  - JCV ELISA negative, or
  - JCV + but no history of previous immunosuppressants, <2 years of Natalizumab
- 1/1000 if
  - Immunosuppressants+ but <2 years
- 5/1000 if
  - >2 years of natalizumab
  - Risk doubles if immunosuppressants history+

10.	EEE Eastern equine encephalitis or sleeping sickness	Rare Fatal Zoonotic disease, caused by Mosquito-vectored Togavirus Suspect in a patient with history of travel to America/USA • Fever + malaise + myalgia • Altered sensorium, then coma • CSF cells ~100	Main question asked in exam is MRI features MRI brain: **PARenthesis sign** • Refers to bilateral FLAIR hyperintensities of Internal capsule and External Capsule • Sparing the lentiform
11.	WNV West Nile encephalitis		Involvement of thalamus and basal ganglia
12.	MVE Murray Valley encephalitis		Involvement of thalamus and basal ganglia Bilateral bulky thalamus

4. PARASITIC INFECTIONS

	Disease	Clinical features	Diagnosis and radiology
1.	Toxoplasma	More common in HIV patients Caused by *Toxoplasma gondii* Due to reactivation of latent cyst in CNS Major cause of morbidity mortality in HIV patients Most common C/P • Headache** • Seizures • FND (focal neurological deficits)	MRI brain • Multiple lesions • Cystic lesions • T2 white/hyperintense • Perilesional edema ++ • Ring enhancement ++ • **Concentric ring sign** • **Eccentric target** sign (see image) Figure 15.8 Contrast brain MRI showing eccentric target sign.
2.	NCC Neuro-cysticercosis	Caused by *Taenia solium*—frequently infects the CNS Initially *Taenia cysticerci* trigger little inflammation; however: • After several years—they degenerate • Then trigger intense inflammation Most common C/P: Seizures* Most sensitive investigation: NCCT* Staging of disease is done by: MRI*	 Figure 15.9 NCCT head and MRI brain showing multiple calcified granulomas.

		NCC	TB
1.	Size of cyst	Small, <20 mm, single mostly	Large, confluent, conglomerate lesions
2.	Margins	Small, smooth margin	Irregular
3.	Perilesional edema	Small, less edema	More edema
4.	Midline shift	Small, less midline shift	More midline shift
5.	Local meningitis	No meningitis	Basal meningitis +
6.	Hydrocephalus	No hydrocephalus	Hydrocephalus+
7.	Nodule	Mural nodule +	No nodule
8.	Location	Present at GM-WM junction	More in posterior fossa, cerebellum
9.	Presence outside CNS	Seen in muscles, orbit, subcutaneous tissue	Seen in chest, pulmonary TB, GIT, lymph nodes

(Continued)

(Continued)

	NCC	TB
10. Spectroscopy	Amino acid peaks	Lipid peak
11. Raised ICP	Raised ICP: Transient	>24 hours
12. MRI T2	T2: Hyperintensity, but Scolex: Hypointense and Eccentric	T2 hypointense Contrast enhancement +
	Figure 15.10	Figure 15.11
13. MRI T1	No T1 hyperintense rim	T1 hyperintense rim on MT-MRI
		Other pointers • **Cranial nerve palsies** • **Vasculitis infarcts** • Lymphocytosis in CSF • High protein, low glucose
		MRI findings in order of prevalence: **Meningeal enhance > Hydrocephalus** > basal exudate > infarcts > Tuberculoma

5. NEUROMUSCULAR DISEASES AND MISCELLANEOUS

	Disease	Clinical features	Radiology and diagnosis
1.	GBS: Guillain-Barré syndrome due to *C. jejuni*	*Campylobacter jejuni* Bacteria Most common cause of AMAN variant in China and Japan AMAN = Pure motor, Axonal GBS	Diagnosis is by nerve conduction studies and CSF analysis CSF shows albumin-cytological dissociation
2.	GBS due to Zika virus	In Zika virus–induced GBS, there is less time between the infection and onset of GBS • **<7 days** • More common in Older age • More common in females • More prominent facial weakness • Cranial nerve deficits	

	Disease	Clinical features	Radiology and diagnosis
3.	Lyme disease	Caused by a Tick bite Suspect in any patient with history • Patient lives near woods • Lives in forest • Patient went on hiking trip	
		Diagnosis is made by characteristic rash After tick bite, the rash develops and clears in 48 hours • However enlarging rash is important Bifacial weakness is common in Lyme Time duration of tick attachment is important Tick attachment <12 hours: Increases the risk of Lyme disease by only 2%	Figure 15.12 **Erythema migrans (EM)**: • Hallmark of Lyme disease • Enlarging painless rash • With Central clearing • Around the site of bite
4.	Botulism	Caused by *Clostridium botulinum* • Serious paralytic illness • Due to Neurotoxins produced by clostridium Foodborne v/s wound botulism (over few days) • Blurring of vision, diplopia • Ophthalmoplegia • Dysarthria, dysphagia • F/b LMN facial palsy • F/b neck and respiratory weakness • F/b arm and leg weakness	Descending weakness is seen in botulism Arm >> f/b >> legs weakness Bilateral weakness, But may be asymmetrical Risk factors for wound botulism • IV drugs • Trauma • Surgery
	Causes of ascending motor paralysis • GBS Causes of descending motor paralysis (face or Upper limb first) • Snake bite • Botulism • Polio • Diphtheria		
5.	LD Labrune disease	Progressive cerebral degeneration Characterized by a triad of • White matter disease (leukodystrophy) • Presence of Cysts in CNS • And Intracranial calcification Cause: SNORD 118 mutation	

INDEX

Note: Page numbers in *italics* indicate a figure and page numbers in **bold** indicate a table on the corresponding page.

A

Abney effect, 33
abnormal visual phenomenon, 31–34
abulia, 2
aceruloplasminemia, 151
acquired neuropathy, 38
acute disseminated encephalomyelitis (ADEM), 87
acute inflammatory demyelination polyradiculoneuropathy (AIDP), 35, 42, 45
  variants of, *43*, **44**
acute intermittent porphyria (AIP), 80
Addison crisis, 80
agrammatic PNFA primary non-fluent aphasia, 110
Alzheimer disease (AD), 104, 109, 111, 114, *115*
  pathology, 113
amyloid beta-related angiitis (ABRA), 3
amyotrophic lateral sclerosis (ALS), 74–75
Andersen–Tawil syndrome (ATS), 60, 61
angioedema, 7
anisocoria, 23, 25
  approach, *24*
anterior spinal artery infarction (ASI), 66
anterior/superior canal BPPV, 83
anti-Amphiphysin antibody encephalitis, 90
anti-DPPX (K channel), 89
anti-DPPX encephalitis, 19
antiepileptic drugs (AEDs), 62, 156
  side effects, 17
anti-GABA-A antibody encephalitis, 90
anti-Hu antibody paraneoplastic syndrome, 91
anti-LG1-encephalitis, 19
anti-MAG antibody neuropathy, **36**
antineutrophilic cytoplasmic antibody (ANCA), **45**
anti-NMDA encephalitis, 19
anti-NMDA-receptor encephalitis, 87–88
anti-Tr antibodies encephalitis, 90
Anton–Babinski syndrome, 33
aphasia, types of, *110*
apperceptive visual agnosia, 33–34
Argyll Robertson pupil (ARP), 25, 26
arteritic-anterior ION (A-AION), 30–31
ASIA scale levels, 70
associative visual agnosia, 34
ataxia telangiectasia (AT), 103
atherosclerosis, 2

autoimmune autonomic ganglionopathy (AAG), 40
autoimmune dementias, 113
autoimmune encephalitis, 87–89
autonomic system neuropathies
  AAG, 40
  PAF, 40
  POTS, 40–41
  transthyretin neuropathy, 41
autosomal recessive spastic ataxia of Charlevoix-Saguenay (ARSACS), 157

B

bacterial meningitis, 167–168
Balint–Holmes syndrome, 33
basal ganglia, 67, 97, 121, 165, 172
  calcifications, 100, 101
  iron deposition, 151
Beçhet's disease, 65, 67
Bell's palsy, 22
beta-propeller protein-associated neurodegeneration (BPAN), 150, 151
Bickerstaff brainstem encephalitis (BBE), 44, 88
bilateral thalamic paramedian infarction, 7
Bing–Neel syndrome, 93
Bolam principle, 86
Bolam test, 86
BotoxA, 137
botulism, 175
Brandt–Daroff exercises, 83

C

C8 neuropathy, 48
CANOMAD, 36
caput medusa, 7
carbamazepine (CBZ), 74, 82, 84, 156
carcinomatous meningitis, 91
carnitine palmitoyltransferase (CPT) II deficiency, 57
carotico-cavernous fistula (CCF), 6
carpal tunnel syndrome, 49
cauda and conus syndromes, 69–70
caudate atrophy, *see* chorea syndromes
Cawthorne–Cooksey exercises, 83
celiac disease, 78
central nervous system (CNS), 87, 93
  autoimmune encephalitis, 87–89
  demyelination disorders, 94